# NON-HODGKIN LYMPHOMA DIET COOKBOOK

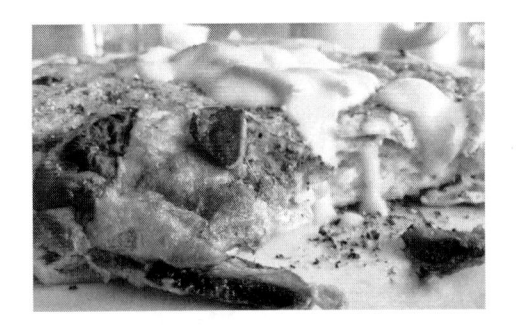

*A Comprehensive Guide for Healing Featuring Cancer-Fighting Recipes and Immune-Boosting Ingredients for Optimal Health and Recovery*

**KELLY C. BROWN**

All rights reserved. No part of this publication may be reproduced, distributed, or transmitted in any form or by any means, including photocopying, recording, or other electronic or mechanical methods, without the prior written permission of the publisher, except in the case of brief quotations embodied in critical reviews and certain other noncommercial uses permitted by copyright law.

Copyright ©[Kelly C. Brown] 2024.

# CONTENTS

**INTRODUCTION**..................10
**CHAPTER 1: UNDERSTANDING NON-HODGKIN LYMPHOMA AND NUTRITION**..................14
    IMPORTANCE OF DIET IN MANAGING THE CONDITION..................16
    FOODS TO EAT AND FOODS TO AVOID.....19
**CHAPTER 2: NON-HODGKIN LYMPHOMA SHOPPING LIST**..................22
    EATING OUT ON THE NON-HODGKIN LYMPHOMA DIET..................25
    7-DAY MEAL PLAN..................28
    Day 1:..................28
    Breakfast: Quinoa porridge with berries and a sprinkle of chia seeds..................28
    Lunch: Grilled chicken breast salad with mixed greens, cherry tomatoes, and olive oil dressing..30
    Snack: Greek yogurt with sliced almonds.......32
    Dinner: Baked salmon, steamed broccoli, and quinoa..................33
    Day 2:..................35
    Breakfast: Whole grain toast with avocado and poached eggs..................35
    Lunch: Lentil soup with a side of whole grain crackers..................37
    Snack: Fresh fruit salad..................40
    Dinner: Stir-fried tofu with colorful vegetables and brown rice..................41

Day 3:................................................................44
Breakfast: Oatmeal with sliced bananas and a drizzle of honey..............................................44
Lunch: Quinoa and black bean salad with a lemon-tahini dressing........................................46
Snack: Handful of mixed nuts.........................48
Dinner: Grilled shrimp skewers with quinoa and roasted asparagus............................................49
Day 4:................................................................52
Breakfast: Smoothie with spinach, kale, banana, and almond milk..................................52
Lunch: Turkey and vegetable wrap with whole grain tortilla......................................................54
Snack: Cottage cheese with pineapple chunks..56
Dinner: Baked chicken breast, sweet potato wedges, and steamed green beans.................57
Day 5:................................................................60
Breakfast: Greek yogurt parfait with granola and mixed berries....................................................60
Lunch: Brown rice bowl with blackened cod and sautéed spinach................................................61
Snack: Hummus with carrot and cucumber sticks.................................................................63
Dinner: Quinoa-stuffed bell peppers with lean ground turkey...................................................65
Day 6:................................................................67
Breakfast: Whole grain pancakes with fresh fruit toppings...........................................................67
Lunch: Chickpea and vegetable curry with quinoa..............................................................69
Snack: Apple slices with almond butter........... 72

Dinner: Grilled trout with quinoa pilaf and roasted Brussels sprouts...................73
Day 7:.........................................................76
Breakfast: Chia seed pudding with almond milk and sliced strawberries....................... 76
Lunch: Spinach and feta stuffed chicken breast with a side of roasted sweet potatoes.............77
Snack: Edamame beans.........................80
Dinner: Vegetable stir-fry with tofu and brown rice................................................... 81

## CHAPTER 3: BREAKFAST................................ 84
Quinoa Breakfast Bowl..............................84
Spinach and Mushroom Omelette...................86
Chia Seed Pudding................................. 87
Greek Yogurt Parfait................................89
Sweet Potato and Kale Hash......................... 90
Salmon Avocado Toast............................. 92
Berry Smoothie Bowl................................94
Cottage Cheese and Fruit Bowl..................... 96
Turmeric Scramble..................................97
Whole Grain Banana Pancakes..................... 98
Almond Butter and Banana Wrap................. 100
Mango Coconut Chia Pudding..................... 101
Green Smoothie................................... 103
Brown Rice Porridge.............................. 105

## CHAPTER 4: LUNCH.......................................108
Grilled Chicken and Quinoa Salad............... 108
Salmon and Broccoli Stir-Fry.......................110
Lentil and Vegetable Soup........................ 112
Turkey and Avocado Wrap........................ 115

Sweet Potato and Black Bean Bowl............. 116
Greek Chickpea Salad................................. 118
Vegetable and Tofu Stir-Fry..........................120
Cauliflower and Lentil Curry......................... 122
Shrimp and Quinoa Bowl.............................. 124
Eggplant and Chickpea Stew...................... 126
Chicken and Vegetable Skewers................. 128

**CHAPTER 5: DINNER..........................................130**
Baked Lemon Herb Chicken......................... 130
Quinoa and Black Bean Stuffed Peppers......132
Salmon with Dill Sauce................................. 134
Vegetarian Lentil Shepherd's Pie.................. 136
Miso Glazed Tofu Stir-Fry.............................139
Cauliflower and Chickpea Curry....................141
Turkey and Vegetable Skillet........................143
Grilled Eggplant Parmesan.......................... 145
Baked Cod with Lemon and Herbs............... 147
Sweet Potato and Lentil Chili....................... 149
Stuffed Portobello Mushrooms..................... 151
Shrimp and Vegetable Skewers.................... 153

**CHAPTER 6: SNACKS AND APPETIZERS......156**
SNACKS...................................................... 156
Greek Yogurt with Berries............................ 156
Homemade Hummus with Veggie Sticks...... 157
Trail Mix with Nuts and Dried Fruit................ 159
Whole Grain Crackers with Avocado............ 161
Cottage Cheese and Pineapple Cups...........162
Baked Sweet Potato Fries............................163
Edamame with Sea Salt...............................165

Apple Slices with Almond Butter.................... 166
Kale Chips........................................................167
Chia Seed Pudding Cups..............................169
Roasted Chickpeas........................................ 170
Cucumber and Tuna Bites............................. 172
Cheese and Whole Grain Crackers.............. 173
Fruit Smoothie................................................174
APPETIZERS.................................................. 175
Guacamole with Veggie Sticks......................175
Quinoa-Stuffed Mushrooms.......................... 177
Smoked Salmon Cucumber Bites................. 179
Greek Yogurt and Herb Dip.......................... 180
Caprese Skewers...........................................181
Roasted Red Pepper Hummus..................... 182
Spinach and Artichoke Dip........................... 184
Sautéed Shrimp with Garlic and Lemon....... 185
Vegetable Spring Rolls................................. 187
Egg White Deviled Eggs............................... 189
Avocado and Tomato Bruschetta................. 191
Cucumber Cups with Tuna Salad................. 192
Zucchini Fritters.............................................194

**CHAPTER 7: SALADS AND DESSERTS......... 196**
SALADS.......................................................... 196
Kale and Berry Salad.................................... 196
Quinoa and Chickpea Salad........................ 198
Spinach and Pomegranate Salad................. 200
Grilled Chicken and Avocado Salad.............201
Cabbage and Apple Slaw............................. 203
Mango and Black Bean Salad......................205

Tuna and White Bean Salad.......................... 206
Roasted Vegetable Quinoa Salad................. 208
Broccoli and Walnut Salad............................ 210
Caprese Salad with Whole Grain Croutons.. 212
Cucumber and Feta Greek Salad................. 213
Sweet Potato and Kale Salad....................... 215
DESSERTS...................................................217
Berry and Yogurt Parfait...............................217
Dark Chocolate-Dipped Strawberries............218
Chia Seed Chocolate Pudding......................219
Baked Apples with Cinnamon....................... 221
Avocado Chocolate Mousse......................... 222
Frozen Banana Bites....................................224
Coconut and Berry Sorbet............................225
Date and Nut Energy Balls...........................227
Baked Peaches with Almonds...................... 229
Pumpkin Pie Smoothie..................................230
Cinnamon-Spiced Roasted Pears................232
Yogurt and Berry Popsicles..........................233
Oatmeal Raisin Cookies...............................234

**CHAPTER 8: HERBS AND SPICES..................238**
Turmeric-Ginger Tea..................................... 238
Garlic and Herb Roasted Vegetables............240
Basil Pesto Sauce......................................... 241
Cilantro-Lime Quinoa.................................... 243
Mint-Infused Fruit Salad................................ 244
Rosemary Lemon Grilled Chicken................. 245
Chia Seed Cinnamon Pudding......................247
Thyme and Lemon Baked Salmon................248

7

Coriander-Cumin Roasted Chickpeas...........250
Dill Yogurt Sauce..............................................252
Oregano and Tomato Quinoa Salad.............253
Sage and Butternut Squash Soup................255
Paprika-Spiced Sweet Potato Wedges..........257
Chamomile Lavender Smoothie....................258

**CHAPTER 9: SOUPS AND STEWS................ 262**
SOUPS.............................................................262
Anti-Inflammatory Turmeric Soup................. 262
Vegetable Quinoa Soup................................ 264
Lentil and Spinach Soup............................... 266
Chicken and Brown Rice Soup..................... 268
Tomato Basil Soup with Chickpeas...............270
Mushroom Barley Soup..................................272
Sweet Potato and Ginger Soup..................... 273
Broccoli and Cheddar Soup.......................... 275
Cauliflower and Leek Soup........................... 278
Bean and Vegetable Minestrone...................280
Spinach and Cannellini Bean Soup.............. 282
Chicken and Vegetable Ginger Soup............284
STEWS........................................................... 286
Chicken and Kale Stew.................................286
Lentil and Sweet Potato Stew....................... 288
Turkey and Bean Chili...................................291
Fish and Vegetable Stew.............................. 293
Cabbage and White Bean Stew....................295
Mushroom and Barley Stew..........................297
Chickpea and Spinach Stew........................ 299
Beef and Vegetable Stew with Turmeric....... 301

Cauliflower and Chickpea Curry Stew...........303
Tomato and Eggplant Stew............................ 305
Black Bean and Quinoa Stew........................ 307
Chicken and Butternut Squash Stew............ 309
Vegetarian Gumbo......................................... 312

**CHAPTER 10: SMOOTHIES.............................. 316**
Tropical Paradise Smoothie.......................... 316
Anti-Inflammatory Turmeric Smoothie...........317
Protein-Packed Peanut Butter Banana Smoothie........................................................ 319
Avocado and Spinach Smoothie................... 320
Golden Mango Turmeric Smoothie............... 322
Basil Berry Delight Smoothie........................ 323
Pineapple Mint Citrus Smoothie....................325
Chia Seed and Berry Smoothie.................... 326
Creamy Almond Butter Date Smoothie......... 328
Beetroot and Berry Smoothie........................329
Cucumber Melon Mint Smoothie...................331
Oatmeal Cookie Smoothie............................ 332

**CONCLUSION..................................................334**
NON-HODGKIN LYMPHOMA DIET MEAL PLANNER...................................................... 336

# INTRODUCTION

Sarah began on a journey of perseverance and optimism after being diagnosed with non-Hodgkin lymphoma. When faced with the difficulties of traditional therapy, she looked for alternatives and discovered the transformative effect of a non-Hodgkin lymphoma diet. Sarah began her healing journey with a fresh emphasis on nutrition, guided by a customized cuisine.

The cookbook, compiled by oncology and nutrition specialists, stressed a plant-based, anti-inflammatory diet high in antioxidants and immune-boosting elements. Sarah accepted her new eating habits, including colorful fruits and vegetables, nutritious grains, and lean proteins in her daily meals. She avoided processed meals, sweets, and harmful fats since she knew how important it was to support her body's natural defense mechanisms.

Sarah discovered the delight of cooking wholesome meals that not only thrilled her taste buds but also powered her body's fight against non-Hodgkin lymphoma with each precisely made recipe. Her nutrition became a source of empowerment for her, giving her a sense of control over her health.

Sarah saw improvements in her overall well-being as she followed the dietary suggestions. Her energy levels soared, and she felt a renewed feeling of life. The cookbook not only gave her recipes, but it also taught her about the science behind each ingredient's possible influence on cancer cells.

Sarah's journey was not without difficulties. Some in the medical community questioned the usefulness of dietary therapies, and she was met with skepticism. Sarah, on the other hand, remained consistent in her devotion to the non-Hodgkin lymphoma diet, armed with a growing body of evidence demonstrating the link between nutrition and cancer.

Her development was observed by regular check-ups and medical examinations, which revealed optimistic signs of improvement. Sarah's oncologist, who was originally skeptical of her alternative approach, noticed favorable changes in her biomarkers and praised her dedication to a better lifestyle.

Sarah's story became an inspiration for others facing non-Hodgkin lymphoma throughout time. Her accomplishment demonstrated the value of a well-balanced, nutrient-dense diet as an adjunct therapy in cancer management. The cuisine that was essential in her journey became popular among patients seeking a more holistic approach to their therapy.

Sarah's resilience, combined with the healing power of a carefully tailored diet, provided a light of hope for individuals suffering similar health issues as the chapters of her life unfolded. Her experience became a testimonial to the transformative power of mindful diet on the path to recovery and well-being.

Welcome to the Non-Hodgkin Lymphoma Diet Cookbook, a comprehensive guide to supporting your body during the difficult road of living with NHL. This cookbook is intended to give a complete selection of dishes aimed to assist persons dealing with the special nutritional needs connected with NHL.

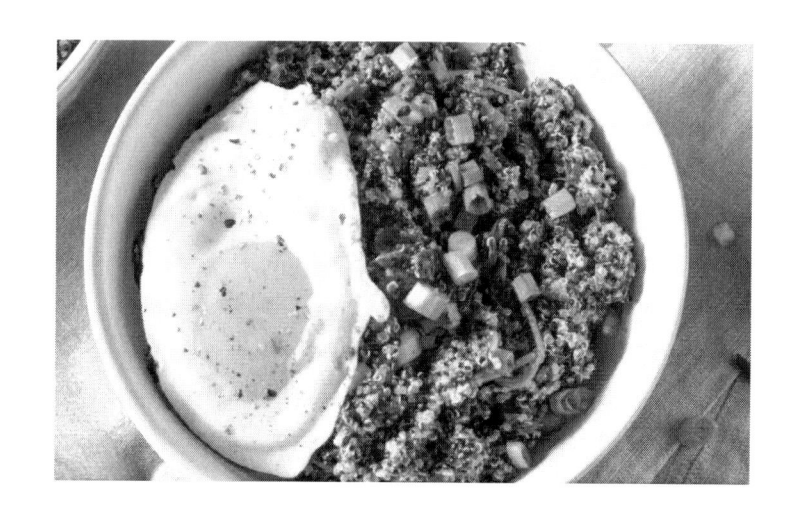

"My commitment to a Non-Hodgkin Lymphoma Diet brings strength to my body."

# CHAPTER 1: UNDERSTANDING NON-HODGKIN LYMPHOMA AND NUTRITION

Non-Hodgkin lymphoma (NHL) is a kind of cancer that begins in the lymphatic system, which is an important part of the body's immune system. As people deal with the problems of this diagnosis, the role of diet in supplementing established therapeutic options becomes more important. We go into the complexities of understanding Non-Hodgkin lymphoma and the dramatic impact nutrition can have on the road to recovery.

1. **Non-Hodgkin Lymphoma and the Lymphatic System:**
   - The lymphatic system, which includes lymph nodes, the spleen, the thymus, and bone marrow, is essential for immunological function.
   - Non-Hodgkin lymphoma is characterized by the uncontrolled proliferation of lymphocytes, a kind of white blood cell that disrupts the normal functioning of the immune system.

- Understanding the kind and stage of NHL is critical for customizing medicinal and nutritional therapies.

2. **Nutritional Issues During Treatment:**
- Patients undergoing therapy frequently experience nausea, loss of appetite, and alterations in taste perception.
- Maintaining a proper diet becomes critical in order to maintain the immune system, prevent malnutrition, and improve general well-being.

3. **The Nutritional Role in Non-Hodgkin Lymphoma:**
- Fruits and vegetables, which are high in antioxidants, play an important role in neutralizing free radicals and promoting immunological function.
- Adequate protein consumption is critical for tissue regeneration, particularly during and after therapies such as chemotherapy.

4. **Mindful Eating for Symptom Management:**
- Tailoring one's diet to treat specific symptoms, such as integrating ginger for nausea or choosing readily digested meals when suffering from digestive troubles.
- Staying hydrated is critical since it aids in the elimination of pollutants and supports numerous bodily functions.

5. **Specialized Diets and Their Impact:**
- Investigating cancer-specific diets such as anti-inflammatory or immune-boosting regimes.
- The Non-Hodgkin Lymphoma Diet Cookbook is a thorough guide that includes recipes that adhere to these dietary recommendations.

## IMPORTANCE OF DIET IN MANAGING THE CONDITION

Non-Hodgkin lymphoma management requires an adequate diet to promote general health and supplement traditional treatments. A specialist cookbook can be a significant resource in this situation, providing recipes suited to the specific nutritional needs of people suffering from this ailment.

1. Nutrient-Rich Diet: A well-balanced diet rich in key nutrients is necessary for patients with non-Hodgkin lymphoma. Recipes in this cookbook include a range of vitamins, minerals, and antioxidants that help the immune system and overall well-being.
2. Energy Requirements: Non-Hodgkin lymphoma and its therapies can have an impact on energy levels. This cookbook includes recipes that supply the calories needed to combat starvation, weariness, and weight loss, assisting individuals in maintaining strength during their health journey.
3. Protein Intake: Protein consumption is essential for tissue repair and immunological function. This cookbook features meals with easily digestible protein sources, which are appropriate for persons experiencing hunger changes or digestive troubles as a result of the ailment or its treatment.
4. Hydration: It is critical for people with non-Hodgkin lymphoma to stay hydrated. This cookbook includes hydrating products and beverages, ensuring that people maintain optimum fluid balance and organ performance.

5. Managing Side Effects: Side effects of treatment, such as nausea, taste changes, or trouble swallowing, might have an impact on dietary choices. This personalized cookbook contains recipes that are intended to ease these negative effects, making it easier for people to enjoy nutritious meals.
6. Immune Support: Non-Hodgkin lymphoma has an impact on the immune system. This cookbook concentrates on immune-boosting components and dishes, integrating meals with immune-boosting qualities to improve the body's ability to fight illnesses.
7. Inflammation Management: Chronic inflammation is linked to cancer, and nutrition plays a role in inflammation management. This cookbook includes anti-inflammatory recipes that emphasize foods with anti-inflammatory qualities to help with general health.
8. Personalized Nutrition: Everyone's dietary requirements are different. A non-Hodgkin lymphoma cookbook can give a choice of recipes, allowing consumers to select meals that match their own preferences, dietary restrictions, and nutritional needs.

# FOODS TO EAT AND FOODS TO AVOID

**FOODS TO EAT:**
1. Fruits and veggies: Eat a range of colorful fruits and vegetables high in antioxidants. Berries, citrus fruits, leafy greens, and cruciferous vegetables like broccoli and Brussels sprouts are examples.
2. Whole Grains: Choose whole grains such as brown rice, quinoa, whole wheat, and oats. These give fiber as well as important nutrients.
3. Lean Protein: Include lean protein sources such as poultry, fish, beans, lentils, and tofu. These contribute to muscle strength and overall wellness.
4. Healthy Fats: Avocados, almonds, seeds, and olive oil are all good sources of healthful fats. These fats supply energy and aid in nutrition absorption.
5. Hydration: Drink plenty of water and herbal teas to stay hydrated. Hydration is critical for general health, particularly during cancer treatment.
6. Probiotics: Consume probiotic foods such as yogurt with living cultures, kefir, and fermented foods such as sauerkraut. These can help with gut health.

7. Herbs and Spices: Herbs and spices such as turmeric, ginger, and garlic can be used. These have anti-inflammatory qualities and may be beneficial to one's health.

**FOODS TO AVOID:**
1. Processed and Red Meats: Limit your diet of processed and red meats because they may increase your risk of cancer.
2. Sugary Foods and Beverages: Sugary foods and beverages should be limited or avoided because they can lead to inflammation and give empty calories.
3. High-Fat Dairy: Choose low-fat or non-dairy options as saturated fats might be harmful to your health.
4. Highly Processed Foods: Reduce your consumption of highly processed meals including chemicals and preservatives. Choose whole, natural foods.
5. Alcohol: Limit or avoid alcohol drinking, as excessive alcohol consumption has been linked to an increased risk of some malignancies.

6. **Excessive Salt:** Limit your consumption of high-sodium foods, which can contribute to water retention and high blood pressure.

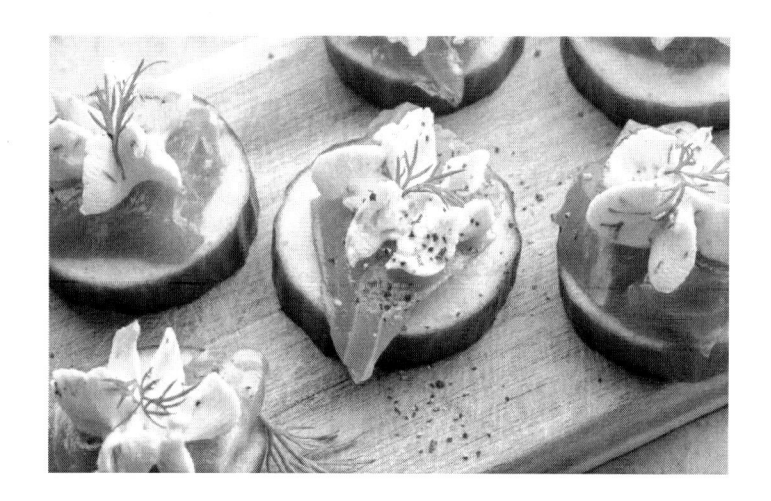

# CHAPTER 2: NON-HODGKIN LYMPHOMA SHOPPING LIST

Making a grocery list for someone with non-Hodgkin lymphoma entails choosing nutrient-dense foods that promote general health and well-being.

**Here's a comprehensive shopping list:**

**Fruits and Vegetables:**
1. Berries: Blueberries, strawberries, raspberries – rich in antioxidants.
2. Citrus Fruits: Oranges, grapefruits, lemons – high in vitamin C.
3. Leafy Greens: Spinach, kale, Swiss chard – excellent sources of vitamins and minerals.
4. Cruciferous Vegetables: Broccoli, cauliflower, Brussels sprouts – provide fiber and antioxidants.
5. Avocados: Healthy fats and essential nutrients.

**Whole Grains:**
1. Brown Rice: A nutritious whole grain providing fiber and energy.

2. Quinoa: Rich in protein, fiber, and various vitamins and minerals.
3. Whole Wheat Products: Whole wheat bread, pasta – for added fiber.

**Lean Proteins:**
1. Poultry: Chicken, turkey – lean protein sources.
2. Fish: Salmon, trout – omega-3 fatty acids can be beneficial.
3. Legumes: Beans, lentils – plant-based protein and fiber.

**Dairy and Alternatives:**
1. Low-Fat Yogurt: Provides probiotics for gut health.
2. Almond or Soy Milk: Dairy alternatives for those sensitive to lactose.

**Healthy Fats:**
1. Nuts and Seeds: Walnuts, almonds, chia seeds – sources of omega-3 fatty acids.
2. Olive Oil: Use for cooking or as a salad dressing.

**Hydration:**
1. Water: Stay well-hydrated to support overall health.

**Herbs and Spices:**
1. Turmeric: Known for its anti-inflammatory properties.
2. Ginger: Adds flavor and has potential health benefits.
3. Garlic: Can enhance the taste of dishes and may have health benefits.

**Probiotic Foods:**
1. Kefir: Fermented dairy product with probiotics.
2. Sauerkraut: Fermented cabbage, a source of probiotics.

**Miscellaneous:**
1. Oats: Versatile and can be used in various dishes.
2. Herbal Teas: Non-caffeinated options for hydration.

**Foods to Limit or Avoid:**
1. Processed Meats: Limit bacon, sausages, and other processed meats.
2. Sugary Foods: Reduce intake of sweets and sugary snacks.
3. High-Fat Dairy: Choose low-fat or non-dairy alternatives.
4. Highly Processed Foods: Minimize packaged and processed foods.
5. Alcohol: Limit or avoid alcoholic beverages.

# EATING OUT ON THE NON-HODGKIN LYMPHOMA DIET

When eating out on a Non-Hodgkin lymphoma (NHL) diet, it's critical to make mindful selections that correspond to your nutritional requirements.

**Here is a restaurant guide to assist you navigate your options while managing or recovering from NHL:**
1. Select Restaurants with a wide Menu: Look for restaurants that have a wide menu with a variety of fresh, whole food selections. This gives you more freedom in selecting things that meet your nutritional needs.

2. Prioritize Lean Proteins: Choose dishes with lean proteins such grilled chicken, turkey, or fish. These protein sources are essential for muscle strength and overall health.
3. Fruits and vegetables should be highlighted: Look for dishes that contain a variety of colorful fruits and vegetables. Salads, steamed vegetables, and fruit-based side dishes can be good sources of important nutrients and antioxidants.
4. Choose Whole Grains: Choose recipes with whole grains such as brown rice, quinoa, or whole wheat alternatives. These grains give fiber as well as other nutritional benefits.
5. Portion Control: Be aware of portion sizes, as larger quantities may promote overeating. To maintain a balanced diet, consider sharing a dish or reserving a portion for later.
6. Request alterations: Do not be afraid to request dietary alterations. Restaurants are frequently willing to accept requests for adjustments such as steaming instead of frying or leaving out specific components.

7. Limit Processed and High-Fat Foods: Avoid overly processed or fried foods. Choose from grilled, baked, or steaming options. Reduce your intake of high-fat foods and opt for better cooking methods.
8. Be Wary of Sauces and Dressings: Many sauces and dressings include significant levels of added sugars and harmful fats. For salads, request dressings on the side and select alternatives such as olive oil and vinegar.
9. Hydration is essential: To stay hydrated, drink water, herbal teas, or other non-caffeinated liquids. Sugary drinks and alcohol should be avoided because they are unhealthy.
10. Plan ahead of time: Before going to the restaurant, look over the menu online. This allows you to plan ahead of time and guarantees you make healthy choices.
11. Listen to Your Body: Pay attention to your body's hunger and fullness cues. Slowly and savor your food, allowing your body time to detect when it is full.
12. Interact with the Staff: Inform the restaurant staff of any special dietary concerns or limits. They can provide ingredient information and assist you in making informed decisions.

# 7-DAY MEAL PLAN

## Day 1:

## Breakfast: Quinoa porridge with berries and a sprinkle of chia seeds

**Ingredients:**
- 1 cup quinoa
- 2 cups water
- 2 cups milk (dairy or plant-based)
- 1 cup mixed berries (strawberries, blueberries, raspberries)
- 2 tablespoons chia seeds
- 2 tablespoons honey or maple syrup
- 1 teaspoon vanilla extract
- Pinch of salt

**Instructions:**
1. Rinse the quinoa thoroughly under cold water to remove any bitterness.
2. In a saucepan, combine the rinsed quinoa and water. Bring it to a boil, then reduce the heat to low, cover, and simmer for about 15 minutes or until the quinoa is cooked and water is absorbed.

3. In another pot, heat the milk over medium heat. Once it's warm, add the cooked quinoa to the milk.
4. Stir in the vanilla extract, salt, and honey or maple syrup. Mix well and let it simmer for an additional 5-7 minutes, allowing the flavors to meld.
5. In the meantime, wash and prepare the mixed berries.
6. Once the quinoa porridge reaches your desired consistency, remove it from the heat.
7. Serve the quinoa porridge in bowls, and top each serving with a generous portion of mixed berries.
8. Sprinkle chia seeds over the berries for added texture and nutritional benefits.
9. Optionally, drizzle a bit more honey or maple syrup on top for sweetness.
10. Enjoy your delicious and nutritious quinoa porridge with berries and chia seeds!

# Lunch: Grilled chicken breast salad with mixed greens, cherry tomatoes, and olive oil dressing

**Ingredients:**

**For the Grilled Chicken:**
- 2 boneless, skinless chicken breasts
- 2 tablespoons olive oil
- 1 teaspoon dried oregano
- 1 teaspoon garlic powder
- Salt and pepper to taste

**For the Salad:**
- 6 cups mixed greens (spinach, arugula, romaine, etc.)
- 1 cup cherry tomatoes, halved
- 1/2 red onion, thinly sliced
- 1 cucumber, sliced
- 1/2 cup Kalamata olives, pitted and sliced

**For the Olive Oil Dressing:**
- 1/4 cup extra-virgin olive oil
- 2 tablespoons red wine vinegar
- 1 teaspoon Dijon mustard
- 1 clove garlic, minced
- Salt and pepper to taste

**Instructions:**
1. Preheat your grill to medium-high heat.
2. In a bowl, mix olive oil, dried oregano, garlic powder, salt, and pepper. Coat the chicken breasts with this mixture.
3. Grill the chicken breasts for about 6-7 minutes per side or until they reach an internal temperature of 165°F (74°C). Let them rest for a few minutes before slicing.
4. While the chicken is grilling, prepare the salad ingredients. Toss together mixed greens, cherry tomatoes, red onion, cucumber, and Kalamata olives in a large salad bowl.
5. In a separate bowl, whisk together extra-virgin olive oil, red wine vinegar, Dijon mustard, minced garlic, salt, and pepper. This will be your dressing.
6. Once the chicken is rested, slice it into thin strips.
7. Add the sliced grilled chicken to the salad.
8. Drizzle the olive oil dressing over the salad and toss gently to coat everything evenly.

9. Serve the grilled chicken breast salad immediately, and enjoy a healthy and flavorful meal!

## Snack: Greek yogurt with sliced almonds

**Ingredients:**
- 1 cup Greek yogurt
- 2 tablespoons sliced almonds
- 1 tablespoon honey or maple syrup (optional for sweetness)
- Fresh berries or fruit slices (optional for garnish)

**Instructions:**
1. Start by choosing a bowl or container for your Greek yogurt.
2. Spoon the Greek yogurt into the bowl, spreading it evenly.
3. In a dry pan over medium heat, toast the sliced almonds until they become golden and fragrant. This usually takes about 2-3 minutes. Be sure to stir frequently to avoid burning.
4. Once the almonds are toasted, let them cool for a minute.

5. Sprinkle the toasted sliced almonds over the Greek yogurt.
6. If you prefer a sweeter taste, drizzle honey or maple syrup over the yogurt and almonds. Adjust the sweetness according to your preference.
7. Optionally, garnish your yogurt with fresh berries or fruit slices for added freshness and flavor.
8. Stir the ingredients gently to combine or leave them layered for a visually appealing presentation.
9. Enjoy your Greek yogurt with sliced almonds as a healthy and satisfying snack or breakfast!

## Dinner: Baked salmon, steamed broccoli, and quinoa

**Ingredients:**
**For Baked Salmon:**
- 4 salmon filets
- 2 tablespoons olive oil
- 2 tablespoons lemon juice
- 2 cloves garlic, minced
- 1 teaspoon dried dill

- Salt and pepper to taste

**For Steamed Broccoli:**
- 2 cups broccoli florets
- 1 tablespoon olive oil
- Salt and pepper to taste

**For Quinoa:**
- 1 cup quinoa
- 2 cups water or vegetable broth
- Salt to taste

**Instructions:**
1. Preheat your oven to 400°F (200°C).
2. Place the salmon filets on a baking sheet lined with parchment paper or lightly greased.
3. In a small bowl, mix together olive oil, lemon juice, minced garlic, dried dill, salt, and pepper. Brush this mixture over the salmon filets.
4. Bake the salmon in the preheated oven for about 15-20 minutes or until the salmon easily flakes with a fork.
5. While the salmon is baking, rinse the quinoa under cold water. Combine quinoa, water or vegetable broth, and a pinch of salt in a saucepan. Bring to a boil, then reduce the heat, cover, and simmer for about 15 minutes or until the liquid is absorbed.

6. In a separate pot, bring water to a boil. Place broccoli florets in a steamer basket and steam for 4-5 minutes or until they are tender-crisp.
7. Drizzle the steamed broccoli with olive oil and season with salt and pepper.
8. Once the quinoa is cooked, fluff it with a fork.
9. Remove the baked salmon from the oven and serve it alongside the steamed broccoli and quinoa.
10. Garnish the dish with additional lemon wedges or fresh herbs if desired.
11. Enjoy your wholesome and nutritious meal of baked salmon, steamed broccoli, and quinoa!

## Day 2:

## Breakfast: Whole grain toast with avocado and poached eggs

**Ingredients:**
- 2 slices whole grain bread
- 1 ripe avocado
- 4 large eggs
- 1 tablespoon white vinegar (for poaching eggs)

- Salt and pepper to taste
- Optional toppings: red pepper flakes, cherry tomatoes, or fresh herbs

**Instructions:**
1. Toast the whole grain bread slices to your desired level of crispiness.
2. While the bread is toasting, cut the avocado in half, remove the pit, and scoop the flesh into a bowl. Mash the avocado with a fork and season it with salt and pepper to taste.
3. Poach the eggs: Bring a pot of water to a gentle simmer. Add white vinegar to the simmering water. Crack each egg into a small bowl. Create a gentle whirlpool in the water and carefully slide the egg into the center. Poach each egg for about 3-4 minutes for a runny yolk.
4. While the eggs are poaching, spread the mashed avocado evenly over the toasted whole grain bread slices.
5. Carefully remove the poached eggs with a slotted spoon and place them on top of the mashed avocado.
6. Season the eggs with a pinch of salt and pepper.

7. Optionally, garnish the dish with red pepper flakes, halved cherry tomatoes, or fresh herbs for added flavor and color.
8. Serve the whole grain toast with avocado and poached eggs immediately, while the eggs are still warm.
9. Enjoy your delicious and nutritious breakfast or brunch!

## Lunch: Lentil soup with a side of whole grain crackers

**Ingredients:**

**For Lentil Soup:**
- 1 cup dried green or brown lentils, rinsed and drained
- 1 onion, finely chopped
- 2 carrots, peeled and diced
- 2 celery stalks, diced
- 3 cloves garlic, minced
- 1 can (14 oz) diced tomatoes
- 6 cups vegetable broth
- 1 teaspoon ground cumin
- 1 teaspoon ground coriander
- 1/2 teaspoon smoked paprika

- 1 bay leaf
- Salt and pepper to taste
- 2 tablespoons olive oil
- Fresh parsley for garnish (optional)

**For Whole Grain Crackers:**
- 1 cup whole wheat flour
- 1/2 cup oats
- 1/4 cup flaxseeds, ground
- 1/4 cup sesame seeds
- 1/4 cup sunflower seeds
- 1/4 cup olive oil
- 1/2 cup water
- 1 teaspoon salt
- 1/2 teaspoon garlic powder (optional)

**Instructions:**

**For Lentil Soup:**

1. In a large pot, heat olive oil over medium heat. Add chopped onions, carrots, and celery. Sauté until the vegetables are softened, about 5 minutes.
2. Add minced garlic, ground cumin, ground coriander, and smoked paprika. Stir and cook for an additional 1-2 minutes until fragrant.

3. Pour in the vegetable broth, add lentils, diced tomatoes (with their juices), and bay leaf. Season with salt and pepper to taste.
4. Bring the soup to a boil, then reduce the heat to low. Cover and simmer for about 25-30 minutes or until the lentils are tender.
5. Remove the bay leaf and adjust seasoning if needed.
6. Ladle the lentil soup into bowls and garnish with fresh parsley if desired.

**For Whole Grain Crackers:**

1. Preheat your oven to 350°F (175°C). Line a baking sheet with parchment paper.
2. In a large bowl, combine whole wheat flour, oats, ground flaxseeds, sesame seeds, sunflower seeds, salt, and garlic powder.
3. Add olive oil to the dry ingredients and mix well. Gradually add water, stirring until the dough comes together.
4. On a floured surface, roll out the dough to your desired thickness. Transfer it to the prepared baking sheet.
5. Using a knife or a pizza cutter, score the dough into desired cracker-sized pieces.

6. Bake in the preheated oven for about 15-20 minutes or until the edges are golden brown and the crackers are crispy.
7. Allow the crackers to cool on the baking sheet for a few minutes, then transfer them to a wire rack to cool completely.

## Snack: Fresh fruit salad

**Ingredients:**
- 2 cups watermelon, cubed
- 1 cup cantaloupe, cubed
- 1 cup pineapple, cubed
- 1 cup grapes, halved
- 1 cup strawberries, hulled and sliced
- 2 kiwi, peeled and sliced
- 1 banana, sliced
- 1 orange, peeled and segmented

**For the Honey-Lime Dressing:**
- 2 tablespoons honey
- 1 tablespoon fresh lime juice
- Zest of 1 lime

**Optional Garnish:**
- Fresh mint leaves

**Instructions:**
1. In a large mixing bowl, combine the watermelon, cantaloupe, pineapple, grapes, strawberries, kiwi, banana, and orange segments.
2. In a small bowl, whisk together honey, fresh lime juice, and lime zest to create the dressing.
3. Pour the honey-lime dressing over the fresh fruits in the large mixing bowl.
4. Gently toss the fruits until they are evenly coated with the dressing.
5. Optionally, garnish the fruit salad with fresh mint leaves for added freshness and aroma.
6. Refrigerate the fruit salad for at least 30 minutes before serving to allow the flavors to meld.
7. Serve the fresh fruit salad chilled and enjoy this colorful and refreshing treat!

## Dinner: Stir-fried tofu with colorful vegetables and brown rice

**Ingredients:**
**For Stir-Fried Tofu:**
- 1 block firm or extra-firm tofu, pressed and cubed
- 2 tablespoons soy sauce

- 1 tablespoon sesame oil
- 1 tablespoon rice vinegar
- 1 tablespoon cornstarch
- 1 tablespoon vegetable oil for cooking

**For Colorful Vegetables:**
- 1 red bell pepper, thinly sliced
- 1 yellow bell pepper, thinly sliced
- 1 carrot, julienned
- 1 cup broccoli florets
- 1 cup snap peas, ends trimmed
- 3 green onions, sliced

**For Brown Rice:**
- 1 cup brown rice
- 2 cups water
- Pinch of salt

**Instructions:**

**For Brown Rice:**
1. Rinse the brown rice under cold water.
2. In a saucepan, combine the brown rice, water, and a pinch of salt. Bring to a boil, then reduce the heat, cover, and simmer for about 45-50 minutes or until the rice is tender and the water is absorbed.
3. Fluff the cooked brown rice with a fork.

**For Stir-Fried Tofu:**
1. In a bowl, whisk together soy sauce, sesame oil, rice vinegar, and cornstarch to create the marinade.
2. Press the tofu to remove excess water, then cut it into cubes.
3. Toss the tofu cubes in the marinade, ensuring they are well-coated. Let it marinate for at least 15 minutes.
4. Heat vegetable oil in a wok or large skillet over medium-high heat.
5. Add the marinated tofu cubes to the hot oil and stir-fry until they become golden and slightly crispy. Remove tofu from the pan and set it aside.

**For Colorful Vegetables:**
1. In the same wok or skillet, add a bit more oil if needed.
2. Stir-fry the sliced bell peppers, julienned carrots, broccoli florets, snap peas, and green onions until they are crisp-tender.
3. Add the cooked tofu back into the wok with the vegetables. Toss everything together.

4. Continue to stir-fry for an additional 2-3 minutes until everything is well combined and heated through.
5. Taste and adjust the seasoning if needed.

**To Serve:**
1. Spoon the stir-fried tofu and colorful vegetables over a bed of brown rice.
2. Garnish with additional sliced green onions or sesame seeds if desired.
3. Serve immediately and enjoy your delicious and nutritious stir-fried tofu with colorful vegetables and brown rice!

## Day 3:

## Breakfast: Oatmeal with sliced bananas and a drizzle of honey

**Ingredients:**
- 1 cup old-fashioned rolled oats
- 2 cups milk (dairy or plant-based)
- Pinch of salt
- 1-2 ripe bananas, sliced
- 2 tablespoons honey

- Optional toppings: chopped nuts, cinnamon, or a splash of vanilla extract

**Instructions:**
1. In a saucepan, combine rolled oats, milk, and a pinch of salt.
2. Bring the mixture to a gentle boil over medium heat, then reduce the heat to low.
3. Simmer the oatmeal, stirring occasionally, for about 5-7 minutes or until it reaches your desired consistency.
4. While the oatmeal is cooking, slice the ripe bananas.
5. Once the oatmeal is ready, remove it from the heat and let it rest for a minute.
6. Spoon the cooked oatmeal into bowls.
7. Top the oatmeal with sliced bananas.
8. Drizzle honey over the oatmeal and bananas for sweetness.
9. Optionally, add chopped nuts, a sprinkle of cinnamon, or a splash of vanilla extract for extra flavor.
10. Stir the toppings gently into the oatmeal.
11. Serve the oatmeal with sliced bananas and a drizzle of honey immediately while it's warm.

# Lunch: Quinoa and black bean salad with a lemon-tahini dressing

**Ingredients:**

**For Quinoa and Black Bean Salad:**
- 1 cup quinoa, rinsed
- 2 cups water or vegetable broth
- 1 can (15 oz) black beans, drained and rinsed
- 1 cup cherry tomatoes, halved
- 1 cucumber, diced
- 1 bell pepper (any color), diced
- 1/2 red onion, finely chopped
- 1/4 cup fresh cilantro, chopped
- Salt and pepper to taste

**For Lemon-Tahini Dressing:**
- 3 tablespoons tahini
- 3 tablespoons extra-virgin olive oil
- Zest and juice of 1 lemon
- 1 clove garlic, minced
- 1 teaspoon maple syrup or honey
- Salt and pepper to taste

**Instructions:**
1. Rinse quinoa under cold water.
2. In a saucepan, combine quinoa and water or vegetable broth.

3. Bring to a boil, then reduce heat, cover, and simmer for about 15 minutes or until quinoa is cooked and liquid is absorbed.
4. Fluff the quinoa with a fork and let it cool to room temperature.
5. In a large bowl, combine the cooked quinoa, black beans, cherry tomatoes, cucumber, bell pepper, red onion, and cilantro.
6. Season the salad with salt and pepper to taste. Toss gently to combine all the ingredients.

**For Lemon-Tahini Dressing:**
1. In a small bowl, whisk together tahini, extra-virgin olive oil, lemon zest, lemon juice, minced garlic, maple syrup or honey, salt, and pepper.
2. Taste the dressing and adjust the seasoning or sweetness according to your preference.
3. Drizzle the Lemon-Tahini Dressing over the quinoa and black bean salad.
4. Toss the salad once more to ensure even coating with the dressing.
5. Let the salad sit for a few minutes to allow the flavors to meld.

6. Serve the quinoa and black bean salad with lemon-tahini dressing chilled or at room temperature.

## Snack: Handful of mixed nuts

**Ingredients:**
- 1 cup almonds
- 1 cup walnuts
- 1 cup cashews
- 1 cup pecans
- 1 tablespoon olive oil
- 1 tablespoon honey
- 1 teaspoon sea salt
- 1/2 teaspoon ground cinnamon

**Instructions:**
1. Preheat your oven to 350°F (175°C) and line a baking sheet with parchment paper.
2. In a large bowl, combine the almonds, walnuts, cashews, and pecans.
3. In a small saucepan, heat the olive oil and honey over low heat until the honey is melted. Stir well to combine.
4. Pour the honey mixture over the mixed nuts and toss until all the nuts are evenly coated.

5. Spread the coated nuts in a single layer on the prepared baking sheet.
6. Sprinkle the sea salt and ground cinnamon evenly over the nuts.
7. Bake in the preheated oven for 15-20 minutes, stirring the nuts halfway through to ensure even roasting.
8. Keep a close eye on the nuts to prevent burning; they should turn golden brown and have a fragrant aroma when done.
9. Once roasted, remove the nuts from the oven and let them cool completely on the baking sheet.
10. Once cooled, break the nuts apart and transfer them to an airtight container for storage.

## Dinner: Grilled shrimp skewers with quinoa and roasted asparagus

**Ingredients:**
**For Grilled Shrimp Skewers:**
- 1 pound large shrimp, peeled and deveined
- 2 tablespoons olive oil
- 2 cloves garlic, minced
- 1 teaspoon paprika

- 1 teaspoon dried oregano
- Salt and pepper to taste
- Lemon wedges for serving

**For Quinoa:**
- 1 cup quinoa, rinsed
- 2 cups water or chicken broth
- Salt to taste

**For Roasted Asparagus:**
- 1 bunch asparagus, trimmed
- 2 tablespoons olive oil
- Salt and pepper to taste
- Lemon zest for garnish (optional)

**Instructions:**

**For Grilled Shrimp Skewers:**
1. In a bowl, combine olive oil, minced garlic, paprika, dried oregano, salt, and pepper.
2. Add the peeled and deveined shrimp to the marinade, ensuring they are well-coated. Allow them to marinate for at least 15-30 minutes.
3. Preheat the grill to medium-high heat.
4. Thread the marinated shrimp onto skewers.
5. Grill the shrimp skewers for about 2-3 minutes per side or until they are opaque and have grill marks.

6. Remove the shrimp skewers from the grill and squeeze fresh lemon juice over them before serving.

**For Quinoa:**
1. In a saucepan, combine quinoa and water or chicken broth. Bring to a boil.
2. Reduce heat to low, cover, and simmer for about 15 minutes or until the liquid is absorbed and the quinoa is cooked.
3. Fluff the quinoa with a fork, season with salt to taste, and set aside.

**For Roasted Asparagus:**
1. Preheat your oven to 400°F (200°C).
2. Place trimmed asparagus on a baking sheet.
3. Drizzle with olive oil and sprinkle with salt and pepper. Toss to coat evenly.
4. Roast the asparagus in the preheated oven for 10-12 minutes or until they are tender-crisp.
5. Optionally, garnish the roasted asparagus with lemon zest for a burst of freshness.

**To Serve:**
1. Arrange a portion of cooked quinoa on each plate.

2. Place grilled shrimp skewers on top of the quinoa.
3. Add a side of roasted asparagus.
4. Garnish with additional lemon wedges for squeezing over the shrimp.
5. Serve immediately and enjoy your delicious and well-balanced meal!

## Day 4:

## Breakfast: Smoothie with spinach, kale, banana, and almond milk

**Ingredients:**
- 1 cup fresh spinach leaves
- 1 cup kale leaves, stems removed
- 1 ripe banana
- 1 cup unsweetened almond milk
- 1/2 cup ice cubes (optional for a colder smoothie)
- 1 tablespoon chia seeds (optional for added nutrition)

**Instructions:**
1. Wash the spinach and kale thoroughly under cold running water to remove any dirt or impurities.
2. Peel the ripe banana and break it into smaller chunks for easier blending.
3. In a blender, combine the fresh spinach leaves, kale leaves, banana chunks, and ice cubes if you prefer a colder smoothie.
4. Pour in the unsweetened almond milk.
5. Optionally, add chia seeds for an extra nutritional boost. Chia seeds add fiber and omega-3 fatty acids to your smoothie.
6. Blend all the ingredients on high speed until the mixture is smooth and creamy. This may take 1-2 minutes, depending on the power of your blender.
7. Stop the blender and scrape down the sides if necessary to ensure all the ingredients are well combined.
8. Taste the smoothie and adjust the sweetness or thickness by adding more almond milk or banana if desired.

9. Once satisfied with the consistency, pour the green smoothie into a glass.
10. Serve immediately and enjoy your nutritious and refreshing spinach, kale, banana, and almond milk smoothie!

## Lunch: Turkey and vegetable wrap with whole grain tortilla

**Ingredients:**
- 1 pound cooked turkey breast, thinly sliced
- 4 whole grain tortillas
- 1 cup mixed vegetables (e.g., bell peppers, cherry tomatoes, cucumbers), thinly sliced
- 1/2 cup red onion, thinly sliced
- 1/2 cup baby spinach leaves
- 1/4 cup feta cheese, crumbled (optional)
- 1/4 cup Greek yogurt or tzatziki sauce
- 1 tablespoon olive oil
- 1 teaspoon dried oregano
- Salt and pepper to taste

**Instructions:**

1. In a skillet, heat olive oil over medium heat. Add sliced red onions and sauté until they become tender and slightly caramelized. Season with salt and pepper.
2. Lay out the whole grain tortillas on a clean surface or plate.
3. Spread a layer of Greek yogurt or tzatziki sauce over each tortilla, leaving a small border around the edges.
4. Place a handful of baby spinach leaves in the center of each tortilla, creating a base for your wrap.
5. Arrange the thinly sliced turkey breast over the bed of spinach.
6. Sprinkle the mixed vegetables evenly over the turkey. You can use a variety of colorful vegetables for added flavor and nutrition.
7. If desired, crumble feta cheese over the vegetables for an extra burst of tanginess.
8. Drizzle a little extra Greek yogurt or tzatziki sauce on top of the fillings.
9. Sprinkle dried oregano over the entire filling for a Mediterranean flavor.

10. To wrap the tortillas, fold in the sides and then roll them tightly from the bottom, creating a secure wrap.
11. Secure each wrap with toothpicks if needed, and slice them in half diagonally for easier handling.
12. Serve immediately, or wrap in parchment paper or foil for a convenient on-the-go meal.

## Snack: Cottage cheese with pineapple chunks

**Ingredients:**
- 1 cup cottage cheese
- 1 cup fresh pineapple chunks (or canned pineapple chunks, drained)
- 2 tablespoons honey (optional, for added sweetness)
- 1/4 cup chopped fresh mint (optional, for garnish)

**Instructions:**
1. In a mixing bowl, spoon out the cottage cheese.
2. Add the fresh pineapple chunks to the cottage cheese. If using canned pineapple, make sure to drain the excess juice before adding.

3. Gently fold the pineapple chunks into the cottage cheese, ensuring even distribution.
4. If you prefer a sweeter flavor, drizzle honey over the cottage cheese and pineapple mixture. Adjust the amount to your taste preference.
5. Once all the ingredients are combined, refrigerate the cottage cheese and pineapple mixture for about 15-30 minutes to allow the flavors to meld.
6. Before serving, give the mixture a gentle stir to make sure the honey is evenly distributed.
7. Optionally, garnish the cottage cheese and pineapple with chopped fresh mint for a burst of freshness.
8. Serve chilled as a refreshing snack, light breakfast, or a healthy dessert alternative.

## Dinner: Baked chicken breast, sweet potato wedges, and steamed green beans

**Ingredients:**
- 4 boneless, skinless chicken breasts

- 4 medium-sized sweet potatoes, peeled and cut into wedges
- 1 pound fresh green beans, trimmed
- 3 tablespoons olive oil
- 2 teaspoons garlic powder
- 2 teaspoons paprika
- 1 teaspoon dried thyme
- Salt and pepper to taste
- Fresh lemon wedges (for serving)

**Instructions:**

1. Preheat the oven to 400°F (200°C).
2. Place the chicken breasts on a cutting board and pat them dry with paper towels. This helps the seasoning adhere better.
3. In a small bowl, mix together 2 tablespoons of olive oil, garlic powder, paprika, dried thyme, salt, and pepper to create a seasoning mixture.
4. Brush each chicken breast with the seasoning mixture, making sure to coat both sides evenly.
5. Place the seasoned chicken breasts on a baking sheet lined with parchment paper or lightly greased.

6. In a separate bowl, toss the sweet potato wedges with the remaining tablespoon of olive oil, salt, and pepper.
7. Arrange the sweet potato wedges on the same baking sheet as the chicken, ensuring they are in a single layer.
8. Bake the chicken and sweet potatoes in the preheated oven for about 25-30 minutes or until the chicken is cooked through and the sweet potatoes are tender, flipping the sweet potato wedges halfway through.
9. While the chicken and sweet potatoes are baking, steam the green beans until they are crisp-tender, about 5-7 minutes.
10. Once everything is cooked, arrange the baked chicken breasts, sweet potato wedges, and steamed green beans on a serving platter.
11. Serve hot, garnishing with fresh lemon wedges for added brightness.

Day 5:

## Breakfast: Greek yogurt parfait with granola and mixed berries

**Ingredients:**
- 2 cups Greek yogurt (unsweetened)
- 1 cup granola (homemade or store-bought)
- 1 cup mixed berries (strawberries, blueberries, raspberries)
- 2 tablespoons honey (optional, for drizzling)
- 1/4 cup chopped nuts (e.g., almonds, walnuts) for extra crunch (optional)

**Instructions:**
1. In serving glasses or bowls, start by layering a spoonful of Greek yogurt at the bottom.
2. Add a layer of granola on top of the yogurt. Ensure an even distribution for a satisfying crunch.
3. Wash and prepare the mixed berries. If using strawberries, hull and slice them.
4. Add a layer of mixed berries over the granola. Feel free to mix and match the berries for a burst of colors and flavors.

5. Repeat the layers, starting with Greek yogurt, followed by granola, and then mixed berries until you reach the top of the glass or bowl.
6. If you prefer a touch of sweetness, drizzle honey over the top layer of berries.
7. Optionally, sprinkle chopped nuts over the parfait for an added crunch and nutritional boost.
8. Repeat the layering process for additional servings if making more than one parfait.
9. Serve immediately and enjoy this delightful Greek yogurt parfait with granola and mixed berries.

## Lunch: Brown rice bowl with blackened cod and sautéed spinach

**Ingredients:**
- 1 cup brown rice, uncooked
- 4 cod filets
- 2 teaspoons blackening seasoning (store-bought or homemade)
- 4 cups fresh spinach leaves, washed and stems removed
- 2 tablespoons olive oil
- 2 cloves garlic, minced

- Salt and pepper to taste
- Lemon wedges for serving

**Instructions:**

1. Cook the brown rice according to the package instructions. Once cooked, fluff it with a fork and set aside.
2. Preheat the oven to 400°F (200°C).
3. Pat the cod filets dry with paper towels. Sprinkle the blackening seasoning evenly on both sides of each filet.
4. Heat 1 tablespoon of olive oil in an oven-safe skillet over medium-high heat. Once hot, add the cod filets to the skillet.
5. Sear the cod filets for 2-3 minutes on each side to create a blackened crust.
6. Transfer the skillet to the preheated oven and bake the cod for an additional 8-10 minutes or until it flakes easily with a fork.
7. While the cod is baking, heat the remaining tablespoon of olive oil in a separate pan over medium heat. Add minced garlic and sauté for about 30 seconds until fragrant.

8. Add the fresh spinach leaves to the pan and sauté until wilted. Season with salt and pepper to taste.
9. To assemble the bowls, spoon a generous portion of cooked brown rice into each bowl.
10. Top the rice with sautéed spinach and place a blackened cod filet on top.
11. Serve the brown rice bowl with lemon wedges on the side for a burst of citrus flavor.
12. Optionally, garnish with fresh herbs like parsley or cilantro.

## Snack: Hummus with carrot and cucumber sticks

**Ingredients:**
- 1 can (15 oz) chickpeas, drained and rinsed
- 1/4 cup tahini
- 2 tablespoons extra-virgin olive oil, plus more for drizzling
- 2 cloves garlic, minced
- Juice of 1 lemon
- 1/2 teaspoon ground cumin
- 1/2 teaspoon paprika (plus extra for garnish)
- Salt and pepper to taste

- 2 tablespoons water (optional, for desired consistency)
- Carrot sticks and cucumber sticks for serving

**Instructions:**
1. In a food processor, combine the chickpeas, tahini, olive oil, minced garlic, lemon juice, ground cumin, paprika, salt, and pepper.
2. Blend the ingredients until smooth. If the hummus is too thick, add water, one tablespoon at a time, until you achieve your desired consistency.
3. Taste the hummus and adjust the seasoning, adding more salt, pepper, or lemon juice as needed.
4. Once the hummus is smooth and well-seasoned, transfer it to a serving bowl.
5. Drizzle a bit of extra-virgin olive oil over the top of the hummus and sprinkle with a pinch of paprika for garnish.
6. Prepare carrot and cucumber sticks by washing, peeling (if desired), and cutting them into manageable sizes for dipping.

7. Arrange the carrot and cucumber sticks around the hummus bowl for a visually appealing presentation.
8. Serve the hummus with carrot and cucumber sticks as a healthy and flavorful snack or appetizer.

## Dinner: Quinoa-stuffed bell peppers with lean ground turkey

**Ingredients:**

- 4 large bell peppers, halved and seeds removed
- 1 cup quinoa, rinsed and cooked according to package instructions
- 1 pound lean ground turkey
- 1 tablespoon olive oil
- 1 small onion, finely chopped
- 2 cloves garlic, minced
- 1 teaspoon ground cumin
- 1 teaspoon chili powder
- 1/2 teaspoon paprika
- Salt and pepper to taste
- 1 can (15 oz) black beans, drained and rinsed
- 1 cup corn kernels (fresh or frozen)
- 1 cup diced tomatoes

- 1 cup shredded cheese (cheddar or your choice)
- Fresh cilantro or parsley for garnish (optional)
- Salsa or Greek yogurt for serving (optional)

**Instructions:**
1. Preheat the oven to 375°F (190°C).
2. Place the bell pepper halves in a baking dish, cut side up. Set aside.
3. In a large skillet, heat olive oil over medium heat. Add the chopped onion and garlic, sautéing until softened.
4. Add the lean ground turkey to the skillet and cook until browned, breaking it into small crumbles with a spoon.
5. Season the turkey with ground cumin, chili powder, paprika, salt, and pepper. Stir to combine.
6. Add the cooked quinoa, black beans, corn, and diced tomatoes to the skillet. Mix well, allowing the flavors to meld. Cook for an additional 3-5 minutes.
7. Stuff each bell pepper half with the quinoa and turkey mixture, pressing it down gently.
8. Sprinkle shredded cheese over the top of each stuffed bell pepper.

9. Cover the baking dish with aluminum foil and bake in the preheated oven for 25-30 minutes or until the peppers are tender.
10. If you prefer a golden-brown cheese topping, remove the foil during the last 5 minutes of baking.
11. Once cooked, remove from the oven and let them cool slightly before serving.
12. Garnish the quinoa-stuffed bell peppers with fresh cilantro or parsley if desired.
13. Serve with salsa or a dollop of Greek yogurt on top, if you like.

## Day 6:

## Breakfast: Whole grain pancakes with fresh fruit toppings

**Ingredients:**
- 1 cup whole wheat flour
- 1 tablespoon sugar
- 1 teaspoon baking powder
- 1/2 teaspoon baking soda
- 1/4 teaspoon salt

- 1 cup buttermilk (or milk with 1 tablespoon white vinegar or lemon juice)
- 1 large egg
- 2 tablespoons unsalted butter, melted
- 1 teaspoon vanilla extract
- Cooking spray or additional butter for greasing the pan

**For Toppings:**

- Fresh fruits (e.g., berries, sliced bananas, kiwi)
- Maple syrup or honey
- Greek yogurt or whipped cream (optional)

**Instructions:**

1. In a large mixing bowl, whisk together the whole wheat flour, sugar, baking powder, baking soda, and salt.
2. In a separate bowl, whisk together the buttermilk, egg, melted butter, and vanilla extract.
3. Pour the wet ingredients into the dry ingredients and stir until just combined. Be careful not to overmix; a few lumps are okay.
4. Let the batter rest for about 5 minutes to allow the baking powder and baking soda to react.

5. Preheat a griddle or non-stick skillet over medium heat. Lightly coat the surface with cooking spray or a small amount of butter.
6. Pour 1/4 cup portions of batter onto the griddle for each pancake. Cook until bubbles form on the surface, then flip and cook until the other side is golden brown.
7. Continue cooking the remaining batter, adjusting the heat as needed.
8. While the pancakes are cooking, prepare your fresh fruit toppings by washing and slicing them.
9. Once all the pancakes are cooked, stack them on a plate and top with fresh fruit.
10. Drizzle with maple syrup or honey, and add a dollop of Greek yogurt or whipped cream if desired.
11. Serve immediately and enjoy your wholesome whole grain pancakes with a burst of fresh fruit flavors!

## Lunch: Chickpea and vegetable curry with quinoa

**Ingredients:**
- 1 cup quinoa, rinsed

- 2 cups water (for cooking quinoa)
- 1 can (15 oz) chickpeas, drained and rinsed
- 2 tablespoons vegetable oil
- 1 large onion, finely chopped
- 3 cloves garlic, minced
- 1 tablespoon fresh ginger, grated
- 1 bell pepper, diced
- 1 zucchini, diced
- 1 carrot, peeled and diced
- 1 cup cherry tomatoes, halved
- 1 can (14 oz) diced tomatoes
- 1 can (14 oz) coconut milk
- 2 tablespoons curry powder
- 1 teaspoon ground cumin
- 1 teaspoon ground coriander
- 1/2 teaspoon turmeric
- 1/2 teaspoon cayenne pepper (adjust to taste)
- Salt and pepper to taste
- Fresh cilantro for garnish (optional)
- Lime wedges for serving (optional)

**Instructions:**

1. In a medium saucepan, combine the rinsed quinoa and water. Bring to a boil, then reduce heat to low, cover, and simmer for 15-20 minutes or until the quinoa is cooked and water is absorbed. Fluff with a fork and set aside.

2. In a large pot or deep skillet, heat the vegetable oil over medium heat. Add chopped onions and sauté until softened.
3. Add minced garlic and grated ginger to the onions, sautéing for an additional minute until fragrant.
4. Stir in the curry powder, ground cumin, ground coriander, turmeric, and cayenne pepper. Cook the spices for 1-2 minutes to release their flavors.
5. Add diced bell pepper, zucchini, and carrot to the pot. Cook for 5-7 minutes until the vegetables start to soften.
6. Pour in the diced tomatoes (with their juice) and cherry tomatoes. Stir well to combine.
7. Add the drained chickpeas to the pot, followed by the coconut milk. Season with salt and pepper.
8. Bring the curry to a simmer and let it cook for 15-20 minutes, allowing the flavors to meld and the vegetables to become tender.
9. Taste and adjust the seasoning as needed. If you prefer a spicier curry, you can add more cayenne pepper.

10. Serve the chickpea and vegetable curry over a bed of quinoa.
11. Garnish with fresh cilantro and lime wedges for an extra burst of flavor.

## Snack: Apple slices with almond butter

**Ingredients:**
- 2 medium-sized apples (e.g., Honeycrisp, Gala), cored and sliced
- 1/4 cup almond butter
- 1 tablespoon honey or maple syrup (optional, for drizzling)
- 1 tablespoon chopped almonds (optional, for garnish)

**Instructions:**
1. Wash, core, and slice the apples into wedges or rings. Arrange them on a serving plate or platter.
2. In a small microwave-safe bowl, gently warm the almond butter until it becomes slightly more fluid. This can be done in the microwave in short intervals or on the stovetop over low heat.

3. Drizzle the warmed almond butter over the apple slices. You can use a spoon or a small squeeze bottle for precision.
4. If desired, drizzle honey or maple syrup over the almond butter for added sweetness.
5. Optionally, sprinkle chopped almonds over the top for extra crunch and texture.
6. Serve the apple slices with almond butter immediately as a healthy and satisfying snack.

## Dinner: Grilled trout with quinoa pilaf and roasted Brussels sprouts

**Ingredients:**
**For Grilled Trout:**
- 4 trout filets
- 2 tablespoons olive oil
- 2 cloves garlic, minced
- 1 teaspoon lemon zest
- 2 tablespoons lemon juice
- 1 teaspoon dried thyme
- Salt and pepper to taste
- Lemon wedges for serving

**For Quinoa Pilaf:**
- 1 cup quinoa, rinsed

- 2 cups vegetable broth or water
- 1 tablespoon olive oil
- 1 small onion, finely chopped
- 1 carrot, diced
- 1 celery stalk, diced
- 1/4 cup chopped parsley
- Salt and pepper to taste

**For Roasted Brussels Sprouts:**
- 1 pound Brussels sprouts, trimmed and halved
- 2 tablespoons olive oil
- Salt and pepper to taste

**Instructions:**
1. Preheat the grill to medium-high heat.
2. In a small bowl, whisk together olive oil, minced garlic, lemon zest, lemon juice, dried thyme, salt, and pepper for the trout marinade.
3. Place the trout filets in a shallow dish and pour the marinade over them, ensuring each filet is coated. Let them marinate while you prepare the other components.
4. In a medium saucepan, heat 1 tablespoon of olive oil over medium heat. Add chopped onion, carrot, and celery for the quinoa pilaf. Sauté until the vegetables are softened.

5. Add rinsed quinoa to the vegetables and sauté for an additional 1-2 minutes.
6. Pour in vegetable broth or water, bring to a boil, then reduce the heat to low. Cover and simmer for 15-20 minutes or until the quinoa is cooked and liquid is absorbed. Fluff with a fork, stir in chopped parsley, and season with salt and pepper.
7. Preheat the oven to 400°F (200°C).
8. Toss halved Brussels sprouts with olive oil, salt, and pepper. Spread them on a baking sheet in a single layer.
9. Roast the Brussels sprouts in the preheated oven for 20-25 minutes or until they are golden brown and crispy on the edges.
10. While the Brussels sprouts are roasting, grill the marinated trout filets for about 3-4 minutes per side or until they are cooked through and easily flake with a fork.
11. Serve the grilled trout over a bed of quinoa pilaf and alongside the roasted Brussels sprouts.
12. Garnish with additional chopped parsley and lemon wedges.

Day 7:

## Breakfast: Chia seed pudding with almond milk and sliced strawberries

**Ingredients:**
- 1/4 cup chia seeds
- 1 cup almond milk (unsweetened)
- 1-2 tablespoons maple syrup or honey (adjust to taste)
- 1/2 teaspoon vanilla extract
- Fresh strawberries, sliced, for topping
- Additional toppings: sliced almonds, shredded coconut (optional)

**Instructions:**
1. In a bowl, combine chia seeds, almond milk, maple syrup (or honey), and vanilla extract. Whisk well to ensure the chia seeds are evenly distributed.
2. Let the mixture sit for 5-10 minutes, then whisk again to prevent clumping. Cover the bowl and refrigerate for at least 2 hours or overnight to allow the chia seeds to absorb the liquid and create a pudding-like consistency.

3. After refrigeration, give the chia pudding a good stir to break up any clumps and achieve a smooth texture.
4. Taste the pudding and adjust the sweetness if needed by adding more maple syrup or honey.
5. To serve, spoon the chia seed pudding into individual bowls or jars.
6. Top the pudding with sliced strawberries, arranging them in a visually appealing manner.
7. Optionally, add extra toppings such as sliced almonds or shredded coconut for added texture and flavor.
8. Serve the chia seed pudding with almond milk and sliced strawberries immediately or refrigerate until ready to enjoy.

## Lunch: Spinach and feta stuffed chicken breast with a side of roasted sweet potatoes

**Ingredients:**
**For Spinach and Feta Stuffed Chicken:**
- 4 boneless, skinless chicken breasts
- 2 cups fresh spinach, chopped

- 1/2 cup crumbled feta cheese
- 2 cloves garlic, minced
- 1 tablespoon olive oil
- Salt and pepper to taste
- Toothpicks or kitchen twine for securing

**For Roasted Sweet Potatoes:**
- 3 medium-sized sweet potatoes, peeled and cut into cubes
- 2 tablespoons olive oil
- 1 teaspoon dried rosemary
- 1 teaspoon paprika
- Salt and pepper to taste

**Instructions:**
1. Preheat the oven to 400°F (200°C).
2. In a skillet, heat 1 tablespoon of olive oil over medium heat. Add minced garlic and sauté for 30 seconds until fragrant.
3. Add chopped spinach to the skillet and cook until wilted. Season with salt and pepper.
4. Remove the skillet from heat and let the spinach cool slightly.
5. In a bowl, combine the cooked spinach with crumbled feta cheese. Mix well.

6. Make a horizontal slit in each chicken breast to create a pocket for stuffing. Be careful not to cut all the way through.
7. Stuff each chicken breast with the spinach and feta mixture, securing the openings with toothpicks or tying with kitchen twine.
8. Season the stuffed chicken breasts with salt and pepper.
9. In a separate bowl, toss sweet potato cubes with olive oil, dried rosemary, paprika, salt, and pepper until well coated.
10. Place the stuffed chicken breasts and sweet potato cubes on a baking sheet lined with parchment paper or lightly greased.
11. Bake in the preheated oven for 25-30 minutes or until the chicken is cooked through and the sweet potatoes are tender, turning the sweet potatoes halfway through.
12. Once cooked, remove the toothpicks or twine from the stuffed chicken breasts.
13. Serve the spinach and feta stuffed chicken breasts alongside the roasted sweet potatoes.

## Snack: Edamame beans

**Ingredients:**

- 2 cups edamame beans (fresh or frozen)
- 1 tablespoon olive oil
- 2 cloves garlic, minced
- 1 teaspoon sea salt (adjust to taste)
- Optional: sesame seeds, lime wedges, or chili flakes for garnish

**Instructions:**

1. If using frozen edamame, thaw them according to the package instructions. If using fresh edamame, remove them from the pods.
2. In a pot of boiling water, cook the edamame beans for about 3-5 minutes or until they are tender.
3. Drain the edamame and transfer them to a bowl of ice water to stop the cooking process. This helps them retain their vibrant green color.
4. Heat olive oil in a skillet over medium heat. Add minced garlic and sauté for about 1-2 minutes until it becomes fragrant but not browned.
5. Add the cooked edamame beans to the skillet, tossing them to coat in the garlic-infused oil. Cook for an additional 2-3 minutes.

6. Sprinkle sea salt over the edamame and continue to toss, ensuring they are evenly seasoned.
7. If desired, garnish with sesame seeds, a squeeze of lime juice, or chili flakes for added flavor.
8. Serve the edamame beans as a snack or side dish.

## Dinner: Vegetable stir-fry with tofu and brown rice

**Ingredients:**
- 1 cup brown rice
- 1 block firm tofu, pressed and cubed
- 2 tablespoons soy sauce
- 1 tablespoon sesame oil
- 1 tablespoon vegetable oil
- 1 onion, thinly sliced
- 2 bell peppers, thinly sliced (use a mix of colors for variety)
- 1 carrot, julienned
- 1 cup broccoli florets
- 1 cup snap peas, ends trimmed
- 3 cloves garlic, minced
- 1 tablespoon fresh ginger, grated
- Salt and pepper to taste

- Green onions, chopped, for garnish

**Instructions:**
1. Cook brown rice according to package instructions.
2. Press the tofu to remove excess water, then cut it into cubes. Marinate the tofu cubes in soy sauce for about 15-20 minutes.
3. Heat vegetable oil in a large wok or skillet over medium-high heat. Add the marinated tofu cubes and cook until golden brown on all sides. Remove tofu from the pan and set aside.
4. In the same pan, add sesame oil. Sauté the sliced onion, bell peppers, julienned carrot, broccoli, and snap peas until they are slightly tender but still crisp.
5. Add minced garlic and grated ginger to the vegetables, stirring continuously for about 1-2 minutes until fragrant.
6. Return the cooked tofu to the pan and toss everything together.
7. Season the stir-fry with salt and pepper to taste.
8. Serve the vegetable stir-fry over the cooked brown rice.
9. Garnish with chopped green onions for added flavor.

"I nourish my body with wholesome ingredients that support my well-being."



"Every meal I prepare is a step towards my health and vitality."

# CHAPTER 3: BREAKFAST

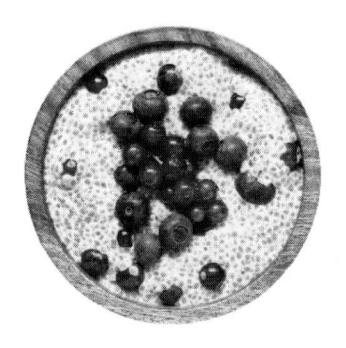

## Quinoa Breakfast Bowl

**Ingredients:**

- 1 cup quinoa, rinsed
- 2 cups almond milk (or any milk of your choice)
- 1 tablespoon honey or maple syrup
- 1 teaspoon vanilla extract
- 1/2 teaspoon cinnamon
- Pinch of salt
- Fresh fruits (e.g., berries, banana slices, kiwi)
- Nuts and seeds (e.g., almonds, chia seeds, pumpkin seeds)
- Greek yogurt or plant-based yogurt
- Optional: drizzle of nut butter or a sprinkle of coconut flakes for garnish

**Instructions:**

1. Rinse the quinoa thoroughly under cold water.
2. In a saucepan, combine quinoa, almond milk, honey or maple syrup, vanilla extract, cinnamon, and a pinch of salt.
3. Bring the mixture to a boil, then reduce the heat to low, cover, and simmer for 15-20 minutes or until the quinoa is cooked and the liquid is absorbed. Fluff the quinoa with a fork.
4. While the quinoa is cooking, prepare your choice of fresh fruits, nuts, and seeds for toppings.
5. Once the quinoa is ready, spoon it into bowls.
6. Top the quinoa with a generous dollop of Greek yogurt or plant-based yogurt.
7. Arrange the fresh fruits, nuts, and seeds on top of the yogurt.
8. Optional: Drizzle a bit of nut butter or sprinkle coconut flakes for extra flavor.
9. Serve the quinoa breakfast bowl warm and enjoy a nutritious and satisfying start to your day!

# Spinach and Mushroom Omelette

**Ingredients:**
- 3 large eggs
- 1/4 cup milk
- Salt and pepper to taste
- 1 tablespoon butter or olive oil
- 1 cup fresh spinach, chopped
- 1/2 cup mushrooms, sliced
- 1/4 cup red bell pepper, diced (optional)
- 1/4 cup feta cheese, crumbled (optional)
- Fresh herbs (e.g., parsley or chives) for garnish

**Instructions:**
1. In a bowl, whisk together the eggs, milk, salt, and pepper until well combined.
2. Heat butter or olive oil in a non-stick skillet over medium heat.
3. Add mushrooms to the skillet and sauté for 2-3 minutes until they begin to soften.
4. Add chopped spinach to the skillet and cook until it wilts, stirring occasionally.
5. If using, add diced red bell pepper to the skillet and sauté for an additional 1-2 minutes.
6. Pour the whisked egg mixture over the vegetables in the skillet.

7. Allow the eggs to set slightly around the edges. Gently lift the edges with a spatula to let any uncooked egg flow underneath.
8. Once the edges are set, but the center is still slightly runny, sprinkle crumbled feta cheese (if using) over one half of the omelette.
9. Carefully fold the omelette in half with a spatula, covering the filling.
10. Cook for an additional 1-2 minutes until the cheese melts, and the eggs are fully cooked.
11. Slide the omelette onto a plate, garnish with fresh herbs, and season with additional salt and pepper if needed.
12. Serve the spinach and mushroom omelette hot, optionally with a side of whole-grain toast or your favorite breakfast sides.

## Chia Seed Pudding

**Ingredients:**

- 1/4 cup chia seeds
- 1 cup almond milk (or any milk of your choice)
- 1 tablespoon maple syrup or honey
- 1/2 teaspoon vanilla extract
- Fresh fruits (e.g., berries, sliced banana)

- Nuts and seeds for topping (e.g., sliced almonds, pumpkin seeds)
- Optional: a pinch of cinnamon or a dash of cocoa powder for flavor

**Instructions:**

1. In a bowl, combine chia seeds, almond milk, maple syrup or honey, and vanilla extract. Whisk the mixture thoroughly to ensure the chia seeds are evenly distributed.
2. Cover the bowl and refrigerate the chia seed mixture for at least 2-3 hours or overnight. During this time, the chia seeds will absorb the liquid and create a pudding-like consistency.
3. After refrigeration, give the chia seed pudding a good stir to break up any clumps and achieve a smooth texture.
4. Taste the pudding and adjust sweetness if needed by adding more maple syrup or honey.
5. Prepare your choice of fresh fruits, nuts, and seeds for topping.
6. Spoon the chia seed pudding into serving glasses or bowls.
7. Top the pudding with fresh fruits, nuts, and seeds of your choice.

8. Optional: Sprinkle a pinch of cinnamon or a dash of cocoa powder for extra flavor.
9. Serve the chia seed pudding immediately and enjoy a healthy and satisfying dessert or breakfast.

## Greek Yogurt Parfait

**Ingredients:**

- 1 cup Greek yogurt
- 2 tablespoons honey or maple syrup
- 1 teaspoon vanilla extract
- 1 cup granola
- 1 cup mixed fresh berries (e.g., strawberries, blueberries, raspberries)
- 1 tablespoon chia seeds (optional)
- 1/4 cup chopped nuts (e.g., almonds, walnuts)
- Fresh mint leaves for garnish (optional)

**Instructions:**

1. In a bowl, mix Greek yogurt with honey or maple syrup and vanilla extract. Stir well until the sweetener is evenly incorporated into the yogurt.
2. Choose your favorite serving glasses or bowls for assembling the parfait.

3. Begin layering the parfait by adding a spoonful of the sweetened Greek yogurt to the bottom of each glass.
4. Add a layer of granola on top of the yogurt. Ensure an even distribution for a balanced taste and texture.
5. Follow with a layer of mixed fresh berries. Feel free to gently press them down to create defined layers.
6. Repeat the layering process until you reach the top of the glass, finishing with a final layer of berries.
7. If using, sprinkle chia seeds over the top for an extra boost of nutrients.
8. Garnish the parfait with chopped nuts and fresh mint leaves for a burst of flavor.
9. Serve the Greek Yogurt Parfait immediately and enjoy this delicious and nutritious treat!

## Sweet Potato and Kale Hash

**Ingredients:**

- 2 medium sweet potatoes, peeled and diced into small cubes
- 2 tablespoons olive oil

- 1 onion, diced
- 2 cloves garlic, minced
- 1 bunch kale, stems removed and leaves chopped
- Salt and pepper to taste
- 1 teaspoon paprika
- 1/2 teaspoon cumin
- 1/4 teaspoon red pepper flakes (optional, for added spice)
- 4 large eggs (optional, for serving)
- Fresh parsley or cilantro for garnish

**Instructions:**

1. Heat olive oil in a large skillet over medium heat.
2. Add diced sweet potatoes to the skillet and cook for 8-10 minutes, or until they start to soften and develop a golden brown crust.
3. Add diced onion to the sweet potatoes and sauté until the onion becomes translucent.
4. Stir in minced garlic and cook for an additional 1-2 minutes until fragrant.
5. Add chopped kale to the skillet. Cook and stir until the kale wilts and becomes tender.

6. Season the hash with salt, pepper, paprika, cumin, and red pepper flakes (if using). Mix well to evenly distribute the spices.
7. Continue cooking the hash for an additional 5-7 minutes, or until the sweet potatoes are fully cooked and tender.
8. While the hash is cooking, you can optionally poach or fry eggs to serve on top.
9. Once the hash is ready, divide it among plates. Top each portion with a poached or fried egg if desired.
10. Garnish with fresh parsley or cilantro for added freshness.
11. Serve the Sweet Potato and Kale Hash hot, and enjoy a nutritious and flavorful meal!

## Salmon Avocado Toast

**Ingredients:**

- 2 slices whole-grain bread (or bread of your choice)
- 1 ripe avocado
- 1 teaspoon lemon juice
- Salt and pepper to taste
- 150g smoked salmon

- 1 tablespoon capers, drained
- 1 tablespoon red onion, finely sliced
- Fresh dill for garnish
- Optional: a drizzle of extra virgin olive oil

**Instructions:**

1. Toast the slices of bread to your preferred level of crispiness.
2. While the bread is toasting, halve and pit the avocado. Scoop out the flesh into a bowl.
3. Mash the avocado in the bowl using a fork. Add lemon juice, salt, and pepper to taste. Mix well.
4. Once the bread is toasted, spread the mashed avocado evenly over each slice.
5. Layer smoked salmon over the mashed avocado on each slice of bread.
6. Sprinkle capers and sliced red onion over the smoked salmon.
7. Garnish each toast with fresh dill for added flavor.
8. Optionally, drizzle a bit of extra virgin olive oil over the top.
9. Serve the Salmon Avocado Toast immediately, and enjoy this delicious and nutritious dish!

## Berry Smoothie Bowl

**Ingredients:**

**For the Smoothie Base:**

- 1 cup frozen mixed berries (strawberries, blueberries, raspberries)
- 1 ripe banana, peeled and frozen
- 1/2 cup Greek yogurt
- 1/2 cup almond milk (or any milk of your choice)
- 1 tablespoon honey or maple syrup (optional, for sweetness)
- 1/2 teaspoon vanilla extract

**Toppings:**

- Fresh berries (e.g., sliced strawberries, blueberries, raspberries)
- Granola
- Chia seeds
- Coconut flakes
- Sliced banana
- Nuts (e.g., almonds, walnuts)
- Drizzle of honey or nut butter (optional)

**Instructions:**
1. In a blender, combine the frozen mixed berries, frozen banana, Greek yogurt, almond milk, honey or maple syrup (if using), and vanilla extract.
2. Blend the ingredients until smooth and creamy. If the mixture is too thick, you can add a bit more almond milk to reach your desired consistency.
3. Pour the smoothie into a bowl.
4. Arrange your choice of toppings on the smoothie. You can create patterns or simply sprinkle them over the surface.
5. Common toppings include fresh berries, granola, chia seeds, coconut flakes, sliced banana, and nuts.
6. Optional: Drizzle a bit of honey or nut butter over the top for added sweetness and flavor.
7. Serve the Berry Smoothie Bowl immediately and enjoy a refreshing and nutritious breakfast or snack!

# Cottage Cheese and Fruit Bowl

**Ingredients:**
- 1 cup cottage cheese
- 1 cup mixed fresh fruits (e.g., berries, sliced kiwi, mango chunks)
- 1 tablespoon honey or maple syrup
- 1/4 cup granola
- 1 tablespoon chopped nuts (e.g., almonds, walnuts)
- Fresh mint leaves for garnish (optional)

**Instructions:**
1. In a bowl, spoon out the cottage cheese, creating a smooth base for your fruit bowl.
2. Wash and prepare your choice of fresh fruits. Berries, sliced kiwi, and mango chunks work well, but you can use any fruits you like.
3. Arrange the mixed fresh fruits on top of the cottage cheese. Be creative and make it visually appealing.
4. Drizzle honey or maple syrup over the fruit for a touch of sweetness.
5. Sprinkle granola over the top. This adds a crunchy texture to complement the creaminess of the cottage cheese.

6. Add chopped nuts for additional crunch and a boost of healthy fats.
7. Optionally, garnish with fresh mint leaves for a burst of freshness.
8. Serve the Cottage Cheese and Fruit Bowl immediately and enjoy a delicious and nutritious snack or breakfast!

## Turmeric Scramble

**Ingredients:**
- 4 large eggs
- 1 tablespoon olive oil
- 1 small onion, finely chopped
- 1 bell pepper, diced (any color)
- 1 teaspoon turmeric powder
- 1/2 teaspoon cumin
- 1/4 teaspoon paprika
- Salt and pepper to taste
- Fresh cilantro or parsley for garnish
- Optional: feta cheese or avocado for serving

**Instructions:**
1. Heat olive oil in a skillet over medium heat.
2. Add finely chopped onion to the skillet and sauté until it becomes translucent.

3. Add diced bell pepper to the skillet and cook until it's softened.
4. In a bowl, whisk the eggs. Add turmeric powder, cumin, paprika, salt, and pepper. Whisk until the spices are well incorporated.
5. Pour the spiced egg mixture into the skillet with onions and bell peppers.
6. Gently stir the eggs continuously with a spatula, allowing them to scramble and cook evenly.
7. Continue cooking until the eggs are fully cooked but still moist.
8. Once the eggs are cooked, remove the skillet from heat.
9. Garnish the turmeric scramble with fresh cilantro or parsley.
10. Serve the scramble hot, optionally with crumbled feta cheese or sliced avocado on top.

## Whole Grain Banana Pancakes

**Ingredients:**
- 1 cup whole wheat flour
- 1 tablespoon sugar (optional)
- 1 teaspoon baking powder
- 1/2 teaspoon baking soda

- 1/4 teaspoon salt
- 1 cup buttermilk
- 1 large egg
- 2 tablespoons unsalted butter, melted
- 1 ripe banana, mashed
- 1 teaspoon vanilla extract
- Cooking spray or additional butter for the pan
- Fresh fruit, nuts, or maple syrup for topping (optional)

**Instructions:**

1. In a large mixing bowl, whisk together the whole wheat flour, sugar (if using), baking powder, baking soda, and salt.
2. In a separate bowl, whisk together buttermilk, egg, melted butter, mashed banana, and vanilla extract.
3. Pour the wet ingredients into the dry ingredients and gently stir until just combined. Be careful not to overmix; a few lumps are okay.
4. Let the batter rest for a few minutes to allow the baking powder to activate.
5. Heat a griddle or non-stick skillet over medium heat. Lightly coat the surface with cooking spray or butter.

6. Pour 1/4 cup of batter onto the griddle for each pancake. Cook until bubbles form on the surface, then flip and cook the other side until golden brown.
7. Repeat the process until all the batter is used.
8. Keep the cooked pancakes warm in a low oven while you finish the rest.
9. Serve the Whole Grain Banana Pancakes with your favorite toppings, such as fresh fruit, nuts, or a drizzle of maple syrup.
10. Enjoy your nutritious and delicious pancakes for a wholesome breakfast!

## Almond Butter and Banana Wrap

**Ingredients:**
- 1 whole wheat tortilla
- 2 tablespoons almond butter
- 1 banana, sliced
- 1 tablespoon honey
- 1 tablespoon chia seeds (optional)
- A sprinkle of cinnamon (optional)

**Instructions:**
1. Lay the whole wheat tortilla flat on a clean surface.

2. Spread almond butter evenly over the entire surface of the tortilla.
3. Place banana slices in a single layer over the almond butter.
4. Drizzle honey over the banana slices for added sweetness.
5. If using, sprinkle chia seeds over the top. Chia seeds add a nutritional boost and a delightful crunch.
6. Optionally, sprinkle a bit of cinnamon over the ingredients for extra flavor.
7. Carefully fold the sides of the tortilla inward and then roll it up tightly, creating a wrap.
8. If desired, you can warm the wrap in a skillet for a minute on each side to make it slightly crispy.
9. Slice the wrap in half diagonally for easier handling.
10. Serve your Almond Butter and Banana Wrap immediately, and enjoy a quick and satisfying breakfast or snack!

## Mango Coconut Chia Pudding

**Ingredients:**
- 1/4 cup chia seeds

- 1 cup coconut milk (full-fat for creamier texture)
- 1 tablespoon honey or maple syrup
- 1/2 teaspoon vanilla extract
- 1 ripe mango, peeled and diced
- 2 tablespoons shredded coconut (unsweetened)
- Fresh mint leaves for garnish (optional)

**Instructions:**

1. In a bowl, combine chia seeds, coconut milk, honey or maple syrup, and vanilla extract. Whisk well to ensure the chia seeds are evenly distributed.
2. Cover the bowl and refrigerate the chia seed mixture for at least 2-3 hours or overnight. Stir occasionally during the first hour to prevent clumping.
3. Once the chia pudding has thickened and set, give it a good stir to break up any remaining clumps.
4. In a separate bowl, combine diced mango and shredded coconut.
5. Take serving glasses or bowls and layer the chia pudding and mango coconut mixture.

6. Repeat the layers until you reach the top of the glass, finishing with a layer of the mango coconut mixture.
7. Garnish the Mango Coconut Chia Pudding with fresh mint leaves for added freshness.
8. Serve the chia pudding immediately, or refrigerate until ready to serve.
9. Enjoy this tropical and nutritious Mango Coconut Chia Pudding as a delightful dessert or a satisfying breakfast!

## Green Smoothie

**Ingredients:**

- 1 cup spinach leaves, washed
- 1/2 cucumber, peeled and sliced
- 1/2 green apple, cored and chopped
- 1/2 banana, peeled
- 1/2 lemon, juiced
- 1/2 cup Greek yogurt
- 1 cup cold water or coconut water
- Ice cubes (optional)
- 1 tablespoon chia seeds (optional, for added texture and nutrition)
- Honey or maple syrup to sweeten (optional)

**Instructions:**

1. Place spinach leaves, cucumber slices, chopped green apple, banana, Greek yogurt, and lemon juice in a blender.
2. Add cold water or coconut water to the blender.
3. If you prefer a colder smoothie, add a handful of ice cubes.
4. Blend the ingredients until smooth and creamy. If needed, stop and scrape down the sides of the blender to ensure everything is well mixed.
5. Taste the smoothie and adjust the sweetness if necessary. You can add honey or maple syrup to your liking.
6. If you want to incorporate chia seeds, add them to the blender and pulse a few times to mix them in without fully blending.
7. Pour the Green Smoothie into glasses.
8. Optionally, garnish with a slice of cucumber or a sprig of mint for presentation.
9. Serve immediately and enjoy your refreshing and nutritious Green Smoothie!

# Brown Rice Porridge

**Ingredients:**

- 1 cup brown rice
- 4 cups water
- 2 cups milk (dairy or plant-based)
- 2 tablespoons honey or maple syrup (adjust to taste)
- 1/2 teaspoon vanilla extract
- 1/2 teaspoon cinnamon
- Pinch of salt
- Toppings: Sliced fruits (e.g., bananas, berries), nuts, seeds, or a dollop of yogurt

**Instructions:**

1. Rinse the brown rice under cold water to remove excess starch.
2. In a medium-sized pot, combine the rinsed brown rice and water. Bring to a boil.
3. Reduce the heat to low, cover, and simmer for about 45-50 minutes, or until the rice is soft and the mixture has a porridge-like consistency. Stir occasionally to prevent sticking.
4. Add milk to the pot, stirring to combine with the cooked rice.

5. Stir in honey or maple syrup, vanilla extract, cinnamon, and a pinch of salt. Adjust sweetness to your liking.
6. Continue to simmer the porridge over low heat for an additional 10-15 minutes, allowing the flavors to meld.
7. If the porridge becomes too thick, you can add more milk to achieve your desired consistency.
8. Once the porridge is cooked to your liking, remove it from heat.
9. Serve the Brown Rice Porridge hot in bowls.
10. Top the porridge with sliced fruits, nuts, seeds, or a dollop of yogurt for added texture and flavor.
11. Optionally, sprinkle a bit more cinnamon on top for garnish.
12. Enjoy this warm and comforting Brown Rice Porridge as a nourishing breakfast or a comforting dessert!

"I am grateful for the abundance of nutrient-rich options available to me."

"Each recipe I explore is a celebration of my dedication to wellness."

# CHAPTER 4: LUNCH

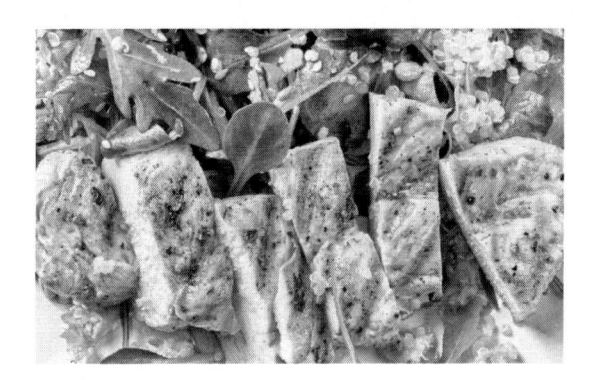

## Grilled Chicken and Quinoa Salad

**Ingredients:**

**For the Grilled Chicken:**

- 2 boneless, skinless chicken breasts
- 2 tablespoons olive oil
- 1 teaspoon paprika
- 1 teaspoon garlic powder
- Salt and pepper to taste
- Juice of 1 lemon

**For the Quinoa Salad:**

- 1 cup quinoa, rinsed
- 2 cups water or chicken broth
- 1 cup cherry tomatoes, halved
- 1 cucumber, diced

- 1 bell pepper, diced (any color)
- 1/4 cup red onion, finely chopped
- 1/4 cup Kalamata olives, sliced
- 1/4 cup feta cheese, crumbled (optional)
- Fresh parsley, chopped, for garnish

**For the Dressing:**
- 1/4 cup olive oil
- 2 tablespoons red wine vinegar
- 1 teaspoon Dijon mustard
- 1 teaspoon honey
- Salt and pepper to taste

**Instructions:**
1. Preheat the grill or grill pan over medium-high heat.
2. In a bowl, mix olive oil, paprika, garlic powder, salt, and pepper. Rub the chicken breasts with this mixture.
3. Grill the chicken for 6-8 minutes per side or until cooked through. During the last few minutes of grilling, squeeze the lemon juice over the chicken. Once cooked, let it rest for a few minutes before slicing.

4. In a saucepan, combine quinoa and water or chicken broth. Bring to a boil, then reduce heat to low, cover, and simmer for 15-20 minutes or until the quinoa is cooked and liquid is absorbed. Fluff with a fork.
5. In a large bowl, combine cooked quinoa, cherry tomatoes, cucumber, bell pepper, red onion, olives, and feta cheese (if using).
6. In a small bowl, whisk together olive oil, red wine vinegar, Dijon mustard, honey, salt, and pepper to create the dressing.
7. Pour the dressing over the quinoa salad and toss to combine.
8. Slice the grilled chicken breasts.
9. Arrange the quinoa salad on plates, top with sliced grilled chicken, and garnish with fresh parsley.
10. Serve the Grilled Chicken and Quinoa Salad as a flavorful and satisfying meal.

## Salmon and Broccoli Stir-Fry

**Ingredients:**
- 1 pound salmon filets, skinless and boneless, cut into bite-sized cubes

- 3 cups broccoli florets
- 1 red bell pepper, thinly sliced
- 2 tablespoons soy sauce
- 1 tablespoon oyster sauce
- 1 tablespoon hoisin sauce
- 1 tablespoon sesame oil
- 1 tablespoon olive oil
- 3 cloves garlic, minced
- 1 tablespoon fresh ginger, grated
- 2 green onions, sliced (for garnish)
- Sesame seeds (for garnish)
- Cooked brown rice or quinoa (for serving)

**Instructions:**

1. In a small bowl, mix soy sauce, oyster sauce, and hoisin sauce to create the stir-fry sauce. Set aside.
2. Heat olive oil and sesame oil in a wok or large skillet over medium-high heat.
3. Add minced garlic and grated ginger to the pan, stir-frying for about 30 seconds until fragrant.
4. Add cubed salmon to the pan and cook until it's browned on all sides. Remove the salmon from the pan and set aside.

5. In the same pan, add a bit more oil if needed, then add broccoli florets and sliced red bell pepper. Stir-fry for 3-4 minutes until the vegetables are slightly tender but still crisp.
6. Return the cooked salmon to the pan with the vegetables.
7. Pour the prepared stir-fry sauce over the salmon and vegetables. Toss everything together to ensure even coating.
8. Cook for an additional 2-3 minutes until the salmon is cooked through and the sauce has thickened.
9. Optional: Adjust the seasoning by adding more soy sauce or hoisin sauce if desired.
10. Serve the Salmon and Broccoli Stir-Fry over cooked brown rice or quinoa.
11. Garnish with sliced green onions and sesame seeds for added flavor and texture.
12. Enjoy your delicious and nutritious Salmon and Broccoli Stir-Fry!

## Lentil and Vegetable Soup

**Ingredients:**
- 1 cup dry green or brown lentils, rinsed

- 1 tablespoon olive oil
- 1 onion, diced
- 2 carrots, diced
- 2 celery stalks, diced
- 3 cloves garlic, minced
- 1 teaspoon ground cumin
- 1 teaspoon ground coriander
- 1/2 teaspoon smoked paprika
- 1/2 teaspoon dried thyme
- 1 can (14 oz) diced tomatoes
- 6 cups vegetable broth
- 2 bay leaves
- Salt and pepper to taste
- 3 cups chopped kale or spinach
- Juice of 1 lemon
- Fresh parsley for garnish (optional)

**Instructions:**

1. Rinse lentils under cold water and set them aside.
2. In a large pot, heat olive oil over medium heat. Add diced onion, carrots, and celery. Sauté for 5-7 minutes until vegetables are softened.

3. Add minced garlic, ground cumin, ground coriander, smoked paprika, and dried thyme. Stir well to coat the vegetables in the spices and cook for an additional 1-2 minutes until fragrant.
4. Pour in the diced tomatoes with their juices and stir.
5. Add the rinsed lentils to the pot.
6. Pour in the vegetable broth and add bay leaves. Season with salt and pepper to taste.
7. Bring the soup to a boil, then reduce the heat to low, cover, and let it simmer for about 25-30 minutes or until the lentils are tender.
8. Add chopped kale or spinach to the pot and stir until the greens are wilted.
9. Squeeze in the juice of one lemon for brightness and additional flavor.
10. Adjust salt and pepper according to your taste.
11. Remove the bay leaves and discard them.
12. Ladle the Lentil and Vegetable Soup into bowls, garnish with fresh parsley if desired, and serve hot.

## Turkey and Avocado Wrap

**Ingredients:**

- 4 large whole-grain or spinach tortillas
- 1 pound thinly sliced turkey breast
- 1 avocado, sliced
- 1 cup cherry tomatoes, halved
- 1/2 cucumber, thinly sliced
- 1/4 cup red onion, thinly sliced
- 4 large lettuce leaves (e.g., Romaine or Bibb)
- 1/4 cup mayonnaise or Greek yogurt
- 1 tablespoon Dijon mustard
- Salt and pepper to taste
- Optional: Sprouts, alfalfa, or microgreens for added freshness
- Optional: Squeeze of lemon or lime juice for extra zest

**Instructions:**

1. Lay out the tortillas on a clean surface.
2. In a small bowl, mix mayonnaise or Greek yogurt with Dijon mustard. Season with salt and pepper to taste.
3. Spread the Dijon-mayo mixture evenly over each tortilla.

4. Place a large lettuce leaf in the center of each tortilla.
5. Arrange slices of turkey over the lettuce leaves.
6. Add avocado slices, cherry tomatoes, cucumber, and red onion on top of the turkey.
7. If using, sprinkle sprouts, alfalfa, or microgreens over the veggies for added freshness.
8. Optional: Squeeze a bit of lemon or lime juice over the ingredients for extra zest.
9. Carefully fold the sides of the tortilla inward and then roll it up tightly, creating a wrap.
10. Slice the Turkey and Avocado Wrap in half diagonally for easier handling.
11. Secure each wrap with toothpicks if needed.
12. Serve immediately, and enjoy this flavorful and nutritious Turkey and Avocado Wrap!

## Sweet Potato and Black Bean Bowl

**Ingredients:**
- 2 medium sweet potatoes, peeled and diced
- 2 tablespoons olive oil
- 1 teaspoon ground cumin
- 1 teaspoon chili powder
- 1/2 teaspoon paprika

- Salt and pepper to taste
- 1 can (15 oz) black beans, drained and rinsed
- 1 cup cooked quinoa or brown rice
- 1 cup corn kernels (fresh or frozen)
- 1 avocado, sliced
- 1/4 cup red onion, finely chopped
- Fresh cilantro for garnish
- Lime wedges for serving

**Instructions:**

1. Preheat the oven to 400°F (200°C).
2. In a bowl, toss diced sweet potatoes with olive oil, ground cumin, chili powder, paprika, salt, and pepper until well coated.
3. Spread the seasoned sweet potatoes on a baking sheet in a single layer.
4. Roast in the preheated oven for 25-30 minutes or until the sweet potatoes are tender and slightly crispy, stirring halfway through.
5. While the sweet potatoes are roasting, heat black beans and corn in a saucepan over medium heat until warmed through.

6. In serving bowls, assemble the Sweet Potato and Black Bean Bowl by layering cooked quinoa or brown rice, roasted sweet potatoes, black beans, corn, sliced avocado, and chopped red onion.
7. Garnish the bowl with fresh cilantro.
8. Serve the bowl with lime wedges on the side for squeezing over the top.
9. Enjoy this delicious and nutritious Sweet Potato and Black Bean Bowl!

## Greek Chickpea Salad

**Ingredients:**
**For the Salad:**
- 2 cans (15 oz each) chickpeas, drained and rinsed
- 1 cucumber, diced
- 1 cup cherry tomatoes, halved
- 1 bell pepper (any color), diced
- 1/2 red onion, finely chopped
- 1/2 cup Kalamata olives, sliced
- 1/2 cup crumbled feta cheese
- Fresh parsley, chopped, for garnish

**For the Dressing:**
- 1/4 cup extra-virgin olive oil

- 2 tablespoons red wine vinegar
- 1 teaspoon dried oregano
- 1 clove garlic, minced
- Salt and pepper to taste
- Juice of 1 lemon

**Instructions:**

1. In a large bowl, combine chickpeas, cucumber, cherry tomatoes, bell pepper, red onion, Kalamata olives, and crumbled feta cheese.
2. In a small bowl or jar, whisk together the dressing ingredients: olive oil, red wine vinegar, dried oregano, minced garlic, salt, pepper, and lemon juice.
3. Pour the dressing over the salad ingredients and toss gently to coat.
4. Let the Greek Chickpea Salad marinate in the refrigerator for at least 30 minutes to allow the flavors to meld.
5. Before serving, garnish the salad with fresh parsley.
6. Taste and adjust the seasoning if needed.
7. Serve the Greek Chickpea Salad as a refreshing and nutritious side dish or a light main course.

# Vegetable and Tofu Stir-Fry

**Ingredients:**

- 1 block firm tofu, pressed and cubed
- 2 tablespoons soy sauce
- 1 tablespoon sesame oil
- 1 tablespoon cornstarch
- 2 tablespoons vegetable oil
- 2 cups broccoli florets
- 1 bell pepper, thinly sliced
- 1 carrot, julienned
- 1 cup snap peas, trimmed
- 3 green onions, sliced
- 3 cloves garlic, minced
- 1 tablespoon ginger, grated
- 1/4 cup low-sodium vegetable broth
- 2 tablespoons hoisin sauce
- 1 tablespoon rice vinegar
- 1 tablespoon mirin (optional)
- Cooked rice or noodles for serving

**Instructions:**

1. Press the tofu to remove excess water, then cut it into cubes. In a bowl, combine the soy sauce, sesame oil, and cornstarch.

2. Add the tofu cubes to the mixture, ensuring they are well-coated, and let it marinate for at least 15 minutes.
3. Heat 1 tablespoon of vegetable oil in a large wok or skillet over medium-high heat. Add the marinated tofu cubes and cook until they are golden brown on all sides. Remove tofu from the pan and set aside.
4. In the same pan, add another tablespoon of vegetable oil. Stir in the minced garlic and grated ginger, cooking for about 30 seconds until fragrant.
5. Add the broccoli, bell pepper, carrot, and snap peas to the pan. Stir-fry the vegetables for 3-5 minutes until they are tender-crisp but still vibrant.
6. Pour in the vegetable broth, hoisin sauce, rice vinegar, and mirin (if using). Stir the sauce and vegetables together.
7. Return the cooked tofu to the pan and toss everything together, ensuring the tofu and vegetables are evenly coated with the sauce.
8. Add the sliced green onions and continue to stir-fry for an additional 1-2 minutes.

9. Taste and adjust the seasoning if needed. If you prefer a saucier stir-fry, you can add more vegetable broth or sauce.
10. Serve the vegetable and tofu stir-fry over cooked rice or noodles.

## Cauliflower and Lentil Curry

**Ingredients:**

- 1 medium-sized cauliflower, cut into florets
- 1 cup dry green or brown lentils, rinsed
- 1 large onion, finely chopped
- 3 cloves garlic, minced
- 1 tablespoon ginger, grated
- 1 can (400ml) coconut milk
- 1 can (400g) diced tomatoes
- 2 tablespoons curry powder
- 1 teaspoon turmeric
- 1 teaspoon cumin
- 1 teaspoon coriander
- 1/2 teaspoon chili powder (adjust to taste)
- 1 tablespoon vegetable oil
- Salt and pepper to taste
- Fresh cilantro for garnish

**Instructions:**

1. Rinse the lentils thoroughly and cook them according to the package instructions until they are tender but not mushy.
2. In a large pot, heat the vegetable oil over medium heat. Add the chopped onion and sauté until it becomes translucent.
3. Add the minced garlic and grated ginger to the pot, stirring for about a minute until fragrant.
4. Add the curry powder, turmeric, cumin, coriander, and chili powder to the pot. Stir well to coat the onions, garlic, and ginger with the spices.
5. Add the cauliflower florets to the pot and stir to coat them with the spice mixture.
6. Pour in the coconut milk and diced tomatoes with their juices. Season with salt and pepper to taste.
7. Bring the mixture to a simmer, then reduce the heat to low, cover, and let it simmer for about 15-20 minutes or until the cauliflower is tender.

8. Once the lentils are cooked, add them to the pot and stir well. Allow the curry to simmer for an additional 10-15 minutes, allowing the flavors to meld.
9. Taste and adjust the seasoning if needed. If you prefer a thinner consistency, you can add more coconut milk or water.
10. Serve the cauliflower and lentil curry over rice or with naan bread. Garnish with fresh cilantro before serving.

## Shrimp and Quinoa Bowl

**Ingredients:**

- 1 cup quinoa
- 2 cups water or vegetable broth
- 1 pound large shrimp, peeled and deveined
- 2 tablespoons olive oil
- 1 teaspoon paprika
- 1 teaspoon garlic powder
- 1/2 teaspoon cumin
- Salt and pepper to taste
- 1 red bell pepper, diced
- 1 yellow bell pepper, diced
- 1 cup cherry tomatoes, halved

- 1 avocado, sliced
- Fresh cilantro, chopped (for garnish)
- Lime wedges (for serving)

**Instructions:**

1. Rinse the quinoa under cold water. In a medium saucepan, combine quinoa and water (or vegetable broth). Bring to a boil, then reduce heat to low, cover, and simmer for about 15 minutes, or until quinoa is cooked and water is absorbed.
2. While the quinoa is cooking, season the shrimp with paprika, garlic powder, cumin, salt, and pepper.
3. In a large skillet, heat olive oil over medium-high heat. Add the seasoned shrimp and cook for 2-3 minutes per side, or until they turn pink and opaque. Remove shrimp from the skillet and set aside.
4. In the same skillet, add diced bell peppers and cook for 2-3 minutes until they start to soften. Add cherry tomatoes and cook for an additional 2 minutes.

5. Combine the cooked quinoa, sautéed vegetables, and cooked shrimp in the skillet. Toss everything together until well mixed and heated through.
6. Serve the shrimp and quinoa mixture in bowls. Top each bowl with sliced avocado, chopped cilantro, and a squeeze of lime juice.
7. Enjoy your delicious and nutritious Shrimp and Quinoa Bowl!

## Eggplant and Chickpea Stew

**Ingredients:**

- 1 large eggplant, diced
- 1 can (15 oz) chickpeas, drained and rinsed
- 1 onion, finely chopped
- 3 cloves garlic, minced
- 1 can (14 oz) diced tomatoes
- 1 cup vegetable broth
- 2 teaspoons ground cumin
- 1 teaspoon ground coriander
- 1 teaspoon smoked paprika
- 1/2 teaspoon cinnamon
- Salt and pepper to taste
- 2 tablespoons olive oil
- Fresh parsley, chopped (for garnish)

**Instructions:**

1. Heat olive oil in a large pot over medium heat. Add chopped onions and minced garlic, sautéing until onions are translucent.
2. Add diced eggplant to the pot and cook for 5-7 minutes until it starts to soften.
3. Stir in ground cumin, ground coriander, smoked paprika, and cinnamon. Cook for an additional 2 minutes to allow the spices to become fragrant.
4. Pour in the diced tomatoes and vegetable broth. Season with salt and pepper to taste. Bring the mixture to a simmer, then reduce heat to low, cover, and let it cook for 15-20 minutes until the eggplant is tender.
5. Add the drained and rinsed chickpeas to the stew. Stir well and let it simmer for an additional 10 minutes to allow the flavors to meld.
6. Taste and adjust the seasoning if needed. If you prefer a thicker stew, you can mash some of the chickpeas against the side of the pot to help thicken the broth.
7. Once the stew is cooked to your liking, serve it hot, garnished with fresh chopped parsley.

# Chicken and Vegetable Skewers

**Ingredients:**
- 1 pound boneless, skinless chicken breasts, cut into bite-sized cubes
- 1 zucchini, sliced into rounds
- 1 bell pepper (any color), cut into chunks
- 1 red onion, cut into wedges
- Cherry tomatoes
- 2 tablespoons olive oil
- 2 cloves garlic, minced
- 1 teaspoon dried oregano
- 1 teaspoon paprika
- 1/2 teaspoon cumin
- Salt and pepper to taste
- Wooden or metal skewers

**Instructions:**
1. If using wooden skewers, soak them in water for at least 30 minutes to prevent burning during cooking.
2. In a bowl, mix olive oil, minced garlic, dried oregano, paprika, cumin, salt, and pepper to create the marinade.

3. Place the chicken cubes in the marinade, ensuring they are well coated. Cover the bowl and let it marinate in the refrigerator for at least 30 minutes, or longer for more flavor.
4. Preheat the grill or grill pan over medium-high heat.
5. Thread the marinated chicken, zucchini slices, bell pepper chunks, red onion wedges, and cherry tomatoes onto the skewers, alternating the ingredients.
6. Brush the skewers with a bit of olive oil to prevent sticking to the grill.
7. Grill the skewers for about 10-15 minutes, turning occasionally, until the chicken is cooked through and the vegetables are tender and slightly charred.
8. Once cooked, remove the skewers from the grill and let them rest for a few minutes.
9. Serve the chicken and vegetable skewers on a platter. Optionally, sprinkle some fresh herbs like parsley or cilantro for added freshness.

# CHAPTER 5: DINNER

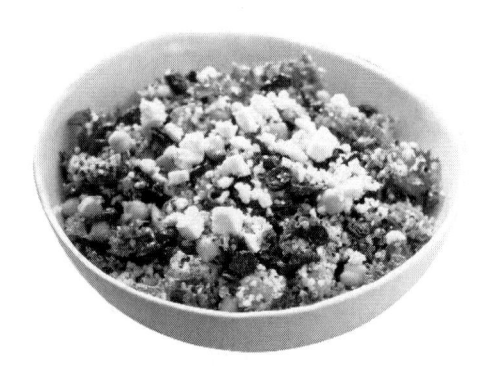

## Baked Lemon Herb Chicken

**Ingredients:**

- 4 boneless, skinless chicken breasts
- 2 lemons
- 3 cloves garlic, minced
- 2 tablespoons fresh parsley, chopped
- 1 tablespoon fresh thyme, chopped
- 1 tablespoon fresh rosemary, chopped
- 1/4 cup olive oil
- Salt and pepper to taste

**Instructions:**

1. Preheat your oven to 375°F (190°C).

2. Start by preparing the marinade. In a bowl, combine the juice of both lemons, minced garlic, chopped parsley, thyme, rosemary, olive oil, salt, and pepper. Mix well to ensure the herbs are evenly distributed.
3. Place the chicken breasts in a large resealable plastic bag or a shallow dish. Pour the marinade over the chicken, making sure each piece is well-coated. Seal the bag or cover the dish and let it marinate in the refrigerator for at least 30 minutes. For a more intense flavor, you can marinate it for up to 4 hours.
4. Once marinated, take the chicken out of the refrigerator and let it come to room temperature for about 15 minutes.
5. Transfer the chicken breasts to a baking dish, arranging them in a single layer. Pour any remaining marinade over the top.
6. Bake in the preheated oven for approximately 25-30 minutes or until the internal temperature reaches 165°F (74°C) and the chicken is golden brown.

7. If desired, you can baste the chicken with the pan juices halfway through the baking time for added flavor and moisture.
8. Once done, remove the chicken from the oven and let it rest for a few minutes before serving. This allows the juices to redistribute, keeping the chicken moist.
9. Garnish with additional fresh herbs and lemon slices if desired.

## Quinoa and Black Bean Stuffed Peppers

**Ingredients:**
- 4 large bell peppers (any color)
- 1 cup quinoa, rinsed
- 2 cups vegetable broth or water
- 1 can (15 ounces) black beans, drained and rinsed
- 1 cup corn kernels (fresh, frozen, or canned)
- 1 cup cherry tomatoes, diced
- 1/2 cup red onion, finely chopped
- 2 cloves garlic, minced
- 1 teaspoon ground cumin
- 1 teaspoon chili powder

- 1/2 teaspoon paprika
- Salt and pepper to taste
- 1 cup shredded cheese (cheddar, Monterey Jack, or a blend)
- Fresh cilantro, chopped (for garnish)
- Sour cream or Greek yogurt (optional, for serving)

**Instructions:**

1. Preheat your oven to 375°F (190°C).
2. Cut the tops off the bell peppers and remove the seeds and membranes. Lightly brush the outside of the peppers with olive oil and place them in a baking dish.
3. In a medium saucepan, combine quinoa and vegetable broth (or water). Bring to a boil, then reduce heat to low, cover, and simmer for about 15 minutes or until the quinoa is cooked and the liquid is absorbed. Fluff the quinoa with a fork.
4. In a large mixing bowl, combine the cooked quinoa, black beans, corn, cherry tomatoes, red onion, minced garlic, ground cumin, chili powder, paprika, salt, and pepper. Mix well to evenly distribute the ingredients and seasonings.

5. Stuff each bell pepper with the quinoa and black bean mixture, pressing down gently to pack the filling.
6. Top each stuffed pepper with shredded cheese.
7. Cover the baking dish with aluminum foil and bake in the preheated oven for 25-30 minutes, or until the peppers are tender.
8. If you prefer a golden, bubbly top, remove the foil during the last 10 minutes of baking.
9. Once done, garnish the stuffed peppers with chopped fresh cilantro.
10. Serve the quinoa and black bean stuffed peppers hot, optionally with a dollop of sour cream or Greek yogurt on the side.

## Salmon with Dill Sauce

**Ingredients:**
**For the Salmon:**
- 4 salmon filets
- Salt and pepper to taste
- 2 tablespoons olive oil
- 1 lemon, sliced (for garnish)

**For the Dill Sauce:**
- 1/2 cup Greek yogurt

- 2 tablespoons mayonnaise
- 2 tablespoons fresh dill, finely chopped
- 1 tablespoon Dijon mustard
- 1 tablespoon lemon juice
- 1 clove garlic, minced
- Salt and pepper to taste

**Instructions:**

1. Preheat your oven to 400°F (200°C).
2. Pat the salmon filets dry with paper towels and season them with salt and pepper on both sides.
3. Heat olive oil in an oven-safe skillet over medium-high heat.
4. Place the salmon filets in the skillet, skin-side down, and sear for 2-3 minutes until the skin is crispy and golden brown.
5. Carefully flip the salmon filets using a spatula and sear the other side for an additional 2 minutes.
6. Transfer the skillet to the preheated oven and bake for 10-12 minutes or until the salmon is cooked through and flakes easily with a fork.
7. While the salmon is baking, prepare the dill sauce. In a bowl, combine Greek yogurt, mayonnaise, chopped fresh dill, Dijon mustard, lemon juice, minced garlic, salt, and pepper. Mix well until smooth.

8. Once the salmon is done, remove it from the oven and transfer the filets to serving plates.
9. Spoon the dill sauce over each salmon filet or serve it on the side.
10. Garnish with lemon slices and additional fresh dill.
11. Serve the salmon with dill sauce immediately, paired with your favorite side dishes.

## Vegetarian Lentil Shepherd's Pie

**Ingredients:**

**For the Lentil Filling:**

- 1 cup dry green or brown lentils, rinsed and drained
- 3 cups vegetable broth
- 1 tablespoon olive oil
- 1 onion, finely chopped
- 2 carrots, diced
- 2 celery stalks, diced
- 3 cloves garlic, minced
- 1 teaspoon dried thyme
- 1 teaspoon dried rosemary
- 1 cup frozen peas
- Salt and pepper to taste

- 2 tablespoons tomato paste
- 1 tablespoon soy sauce (optional, for added depth of flavor)
- 2 tablespoons all-purpose flour (or a gluten-free alternative)
- 1 cup vegetable broth (additional, for the flour mixture)

**For the Mashed Potato Topping:**
- 4 large potatoes, peeled and diced
- 1/2 cup unsweetened almond milk (or any milk of your choice)
- 2 tablespoons vegan butter
- Salt and pepper to taste

**Instructions:**
1. Preheat your oven to 400°F (200°C).
2. In a medium saucepan, combine lentils and 3 cups of vegetable broth. Bring to a boil, then reduce heat to low, cover, and simmer for about 20-25 minutes or until lentils are tender but not mushy. Drain any excess liquid.
3. While the lentils are cooking, prepare the mashed potato topping. Boil the peeled and diced potatoes in a large pot of salted water until tender. Drain and mash the potatoes with almond milk, vegan butter, salt, and pepper until smooth. Set aside.

4. In a large skillet, heat olive oil over medium heat. Add chopped onion, carrots, and celery. Sauté for about 5 minutes until the vegetables start to soften.
5. Add minced garlic, thyme, rosemary, frozen peas, salt, and pepper to the skillet. Stir and cook for an additional 2-3 minutes.
6. Stir in the cooked lentils, tomato paste, and soy sauce (if using). Cook for another 2-3 minutes.
7. In a small bowl, whisk together the flour and 1 cup of vegetable broth until smooth. Pour this mixture into the lentil and vegetable mixture, stirring continuously until the mixture thickens. Remove from heat.
8. Transfer the lentil filling to a baking dish and spread it evenly.
9. Spoon the mashed potatoes over the lentil filling, spreading them to cover the entire surface.
10. Use a fork to create a decorative pattern on the mashed potato topping.
11. Bake in the preheated oven for 20-25 minutes or until the top is golden brown.

12. Allow the Vegetarian Lentil Shepherd's Pie to cool for a few minutes before serving.

## Miso Glazed Tofu Stir-Fry

**Ingredients:**

- 1 block firm tofu, pressed and cubed
- 3 tablespoons white miso paste
- 2 tablespoons soy sauce
- 1 tablespoon rice vinegar
- 1 tablespoon mirin
- 1 tablespoon sesame oil
- 1 tablespoon maple syrup or agave nectar
- 2 tablespoons vegetable oil
- 2 cups broccoli florets
- 1 bell pepper, thinly sliced
- 1 carrot, julienned
- 1 cup snap peas, trimmed
- 3 cloves garlic, minced
- 1 tablespoon ginger, grated
- Cooked brown rice or noodles for serving
- Sesame seeds and sliced green onions for garnish

**Instructions:**

1. Press the tofu to remove excess water, then cut it into cubes. In a bowl, whisk together the white miso paste, soy sauce, rice vinegar, mirin, sesame oil, and maple syrup/agave nectar. Add the tofu cubes to the mixture, ensuring they are well-coated, and let it marinate for at least 15 minutes.
2. Heat 1 tablespoon of vegetable oil in a large wok or skillet over medium-high heat. Add the marinated tofu cubes and cook until they are golden brown on all sides. Remove tofu from the pan and set aside.
3. In the same pan, add another tablespoon of vegetable oil. Stir in the minced garlic and grated ginger, cooking for about 30 seconds until fragrant.
4. Add the broccoli, bell pepper, carrot, and snap peas to the pan. Stir-fry the vegetables for 3-5 minutes until they are tender-crisp but still vibrant.
5. Return the cooked tofu to the pan with the vegetables.

6. Pour any remaining marinade over the tofu and vegetables. Toss everything together, ensuring the tofu and vegetables are evenly coated with the miso glaze.
7. Cook for an additional 2-3 minutes until everything is heated through.
8. Serve the Miso Glazed Tofu Stir-Fry over cooked brown rice or noodles.
9. Garnish with sesame seeds and sliced green onions.

## Cauliflower and Chickpea Curry

**Ingredients:**
- 1 medium-sized cauliflower, cut into florets
- 1 can (15 oz) chickpeas, drained and rinsed
- 1 large onion, finely chopped
- 3 cloves garlic, minced
- 1 tablespoon ginger, grated
- 1 can (400ml) coconut milk
- 1 can (400g) diced tomatoes
- 2 tablespoons curry powder
- 1 teaspoon turmeric
- 1 teaspoon cumin
- 1 teaspoon coriander

- 1/2 teaspoon cayenne pepper (optional, for heat)
- 1 tablespoon vegetable oil
- Salt and pepper to taste
- Fresh cilantro for garnish
- Cooked basmati rice or naan bread for serving

**Instructions:**
1. In a large pot, heat the vegetable oil over medium heat. Add the chopped onion and sauté until it becomes translucent.
2. Add the minced garlic and grated ginger to the pot, stirring for about a minute until fragrant.
3. Add the curry powder, turmeric, cumin, coriander, and cayenne pepper (if using) to the pot. Stir well to coat the onions, garlic, and ginger with the spices.
4. Add the cauliflower florets to the pot and stir to coat them with the spice mixture.
5. Pour in the coconut milk and diced tomatoes with their juices. Season with salt and pepper to taste.
6. Bring the mixture to a simmer, then reduce the heat to low, cover, and let it simmer for about 15-20 minutes or until the cauliflower is tender.

7. Add the chickpeas to the pot and stir well. Allow the curry to simmer for an additional 10-15 minutes, allowing the flavors to meld.
8. Taste and adjust the seasoning if needed. If you prefer a thinner consistency, you can add more coconut milk or water.
9. Serve the Cauliflower and Chickpea Curry over cooked basmati rice or with naan bread.
10. Garnish with fresh cilantro before serving.

## Turkey and Vegetable Skillet

**Ingredients:**
- 1 pound ground turkey
- 1 tablespoon olive oil
- 1 large onion, finely chopped
- 2 bell peppers, diced (any color)
- 1 zucchini, diced
- 2 carrots, peeled and diced
- 3 cloves garlic, minced
- 1 teaspoon dried oregano
- 1 teaspoon dried basil
- 1 teaspoon ground cumin
- 1 teaspoon paprika
- Salt and pepper to taste

- 1 can (14 oz) diced tomatoes
- 1 cup corn kernels (fresh, frozen, or canned)
- 1 cup cooked quinoa or rice
- Fresh parsley for garnish (optional)

**Instructions:**

1. In a large skillet, heat olive oil over medium-high heat. Add ground turkey and cook until browned, breaking it apart with a spoon as it cooks.
2. Add chopped onion to the skillet and cook until softened, about 3-5 minutes.
3. Stir in diced bell peppers, zucchini, and carrots. Cook for another 5-7 minutes until the vegetables begin to soften.
4. Add minced garlic, dried oregano, dried basil, ground cumin, paprika, salt, and pepper. Stir well to combine and let the spices cook for about 1-2 minutes until fragrant.
5. Pour in the diced tomatoes (with their juices) and corn kernels. Stir the mixture and let it simmer for 10-15 minutes, allowing the flavors to meld.
6. Add the cooked quinoa or rice to the skillet, stirring to combine and heat through.

7. Taste and adjust the seasoning if needed.
8. Garnish with fresh parsley if desired.
9. Serve the Turkey and Vegetable Skillet hot, and enjoy a nutritious and flavorful meal!

## Grilled Eggplant Parmesan

**Ingredients:**
- 2 large eggplants, sliced into 1/2-inch rounds
- Salt for sweating the eggplant
- Olive oil for brushing
- 2 cups marinara sauce (store-bought or homemade)
- 1 cup shredded mozzarella cheese
- 1/2 cup grated Parmesan cheese
- 1/2 cup breadcrumbs
- 1/4 cup fresh basil, chopped
- 1/4 cup fresh parsley, chopped
- 2 cloves garlic, minced
- Salt and pepper to taste

**Instructions:**
1. Slice the eggplants into 1/2-inch rounds. Sprinkle both sides of each round with salt and place them in a colander to sweat for about 30 minutes. This helps remove excess moisture and bitterness.

2. Preheat your grill to medium-high heat.
3. After sweating, rinse the eggplant slices under cold water and pat them dry with a paper towel.
4. Brush the eggplant slices with olive oil on both sides.
5. Grill the eggplant slices for 2-3 minutes per side or until they have nice grill marks and are tender. Remove them from the grill and set aside.
6. In a bowl, combine the breadcrumbs, grated Parmesan, chopped basil, chopped parsley, minced garlic, salt, and pepper. Mix well to create the breadcrumb mixture.
7. Preheat your oven to 375°F (190°C).
8. In a baking dish, spread a thin layer of marinara sauce.
9. Arrange a layer of grilled eggplant slices on top of the sauce.
10. Sprinkle a portion of the breadcrumb mixture over the eggplant slices, followed by a layer of shredded mozzarella.
11. Repeat the layers, finishing with a generous layer of mozzarella on top.

12. Bake in the preheated oven for 25-30 minutes or until the cheese is melted and bubbly, and the top is golden brown.
13. Remove from the oven and let it rest for a few minutes before serving.
14. Garnish with additional fresh basil or parsley if desired.

## Baked Cod with Lemon and Herbs

**Ingredients:**
- 4 cod filets (about 6 ounces each)
- Salt and black pepper to taste
- 2 tablespoons olive oil
- 2 tablespoons fresh lemon juice
- 2 teaspoons Dijon mustard
- 2 cloves garlic, minced
- 1 teaspoon dried oregano
- 1 teaspoon dried thyme
- 1 teaspoon dried rosemary
- Zest of 1 lemon
- Lemon slices for garnish
- Fresh parsley, chopped, for garnish

**Instructions:**
1. Preheat your oven to 400°F (200°C).

2. Pat the cod filets dry with paper towels and season both sides with salt and black pepper.
3. In a small bowl, whisk together olive oil, lemon juice, Dijon mustard, minced garlic, dried oregano, dried thyme, dried rosemary, and lemon zest. This creates the marinade.
4. Place the cod filets in a shallow dish and pour the marinade over them, ensuring each filet is coated. Let them marinate for about 15-20 minutes.
5. Line a baking dish with parchment paper or lightly grease it.
6. Transfer the cod filets to the prepared baking dish, arranging them in a single layer.
7. Drizzle any remaining marinade over the filets.
8. Bake in the preheated oven for 12-15 minutes or until the cod is opaque and easily flakes with a fork.
9. If desired, broil for an additional 1-2 minutes to achieve a golden-brown top.
10. Garnish with lemon slices and chopped fresh parsley.

11. Serve the Baked Cod with Lemon and Herbs over a bed of steamed vegetables, rice, or quinoa.

## Sweet Potato and Lentil Chili

**Ingredients:**

- 1 cup dry green or brown lentils, rinsed
- 2 large sweet potatoes, peeled and diced
- 1 tablespoon olive oil
- 1 large onion, finely chopped
- 3 cloves garlic, minced
- 1 red bell pepper, diced
- 1 yellow bell pepper, diced
- 1 can (14 oz) diced tomatoes
- 1 can (15 oz) black beans, drained and rinsed
- 1 can (15 oz) kidney beans, drained and rinsed
- 4 cups vegetable broth
- 2 tablespoons tomato paste
- 2 tablespoons chili powder
- 1 teaspoon cumin
- 1 teaspoon paprika
- 1/2 teaspoon cinnamon
- Salt and black pepper to taste
- Juice of 1 lime

- Fresh cilantro for garnish
- Avocado slices for topping (optional)

**Instructions:**

1. In a large pot, heat olive oil over medium heat. Add the chopped onion and sauté until it becomes translucent.
2. Add minced garlic and diced sweet potatoes to the pot, stirring for about 5 minutes until the sweet potatoes begin to soften.
3. Stir in the diced red and yellow bell peppers, continuing to sauté for an additional 3-5 minutes.
4. Add chili powder, cumin, paprika, cinnamon, salt, and black pepper. Stir well to coat the vegetables with the spices.
5. Pour in the vegetable broth, diced tomatoes, black beans, kidney beans, lentils, and tomato paste. Bring the mixture to a boil.
6. Reduce the heat to low, cover the pot, and let it simmer for about 25-30 minutes or until the lentils and sweet potatoes are tender.
7. Stir in the lime juice and adjust the seasoning if needed.

8. Serve the Sweet Potato and Lentil Chili hot, garnished with fresh cilantro and topped with avocado slices if desired.

## Stuffed Portobello Mushrooms

**Ingredients:**
- 4 large portobello mushrooms, stems removed
- 2 tablespoons olive oil
- 1 onion, finely chopped
- 2 cloves garlic, minced
- 1 red bell pepper, diced
- 1 yellow bell pepper, diced
- 1 cup spinach, chopped
- 1 cup cherry tomatoes, halved
- 1 cup cooked quinoa or rice
- 1/2 cup feta cheese, crumbled
- 1/4 cup fresh basil, chopped
- Salt and black pepper to taste
- Balsamic glaze for drizzling (optional)
- Fresh parsley for garnish

**Instructions:**
1. Preheat your oven to 375°F (190°C).

2. Clean the portobello mushrooms and remove the stems. Lightly brush the mushroom caps with olive oil and place them on a baking sheet.
3. In a large skillet, heat 1 tablespoon of olive oil over medium heat. Add the chopped onion and sauté until it becomes translucent.
4. Add minced garlic and diced bell peppers to the skillet, stirring for about 3-5 minutes until the vegetables are tender.
5. Stir in chopped spinach and cook for an additional 2 minutes until it wilts.
6. Remove the skillet from the heat and add cherry tomatoes, cooked quinoa or rice, feta cheese, and chopped basil. Mix well to combine.
7. Season the stuffing mixture with salt and black pepper to taste.
8. Spoon the stuffing into the portobello mushroom caps, pressing it down gently.
9. Bake in the preheated oven for 20-25 minutes or until the mushrooms are tender and the stuffing is heated through.
10. Optional: Drizzle balsamic glaze over the stuffed mushrooms for added flavor.
11. Garnish with fresh parsley before serving.

12. Serve the Stuffed Portobello Mushrooms as a delicious and satisfying vegetarian main dish.

## Shrimp and Vegetable Skewers

**Ingredients:**

- 1 pound large shrimp, peeled and deveined
- 1 zucchini, sliced into rounds
- 1 bell pepper, cut into chunks (any color)
- 1 red onion, cut into chunks
- Cherry tomatoes
- 1/4 cup olive oil
- 3 tablespoons lemon juice
- 2 cloves garlic, minced
- 1 teaspoon dried oregano
- 1 teaspoon dried thyme
- 1 teaspoon paprika
- Salt and black pepper to taste
- Wooden skewers, soaked in water for 30 minutes
- Lemon wedges for serving
- Fresh parsley for garnish

**Instructions:**
1. In a bowl, whisk together olive oil, lemon juice, minced garlic, dried oregano, dried thyme, paprika, salt, and black pepper. This creates the marinade.
2. Place the shrimp in a shallow dish and pour half of the marinade over them. Toss to coat the shrimp evenly and let them marinate for about 15-20 minutes.
3. In a separate bowl, toss the zucchini, bell pepper chunks, red onion chunks, and cherry tomatoes with the remaining marinade. Ensure the vegetables are well-coated.
4. Preheat your grill to medium-high heat.
5. Thread the marinated shrimp, zucchini, bell pepper, red onion, and cherry tomatoes onto the soaked wooden skewers, alternating ingredients.
6. Grill the skewers for 2-3 minutes per side or until the shrimp are opaque and the vegetables have nice grill marks.
7. Remove the skewers from the grill and transfer them to a serving platter.
8. Optional: Squeeze fresh lemon juice over the skewers for extra brightness.

9. Garnish with fresh parsley and serve the Shrimp and Vegetable Skewers immediately.
10. Enjoy your delicious and colorful grilled skewers as a delightful and healthy meal!

## "My kitchen is a space of positive energy and healing intentions."

## "I am in control of my health, and my choices reflect that power."

# CHAPTER 6: SNACKS AND APPETIZERS

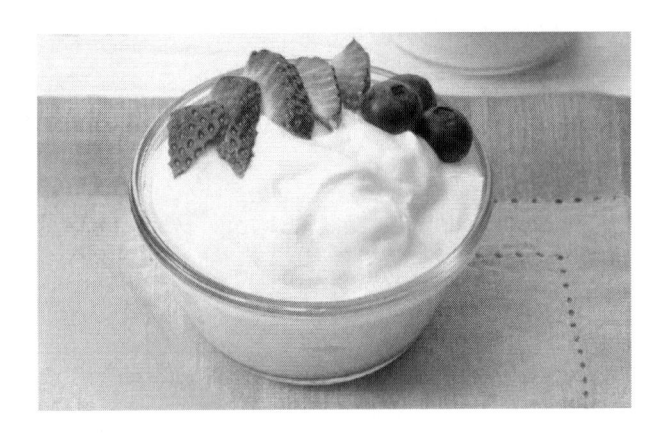

## SNACKS

## Greek Yogurt with Berries

**Ingredients:**

- 1 cup Greek yogurt (full-fat or low-fat, as per preference)
- 1 cup mixed berries (strawberries, blueberries, raspberries)
- 1 tablespoon honey or maple syrup (optional, for sweetness)
- 1/4 cup granola (optional, for crunch)
- Fresh mint leaves for garnish (optional)

**Instructions:**

1. In a serving bowl or individual bowls, spoon the Greek yogurt.
2. Wash and prepare the mixed berries. If using strawberries, hull and slice them.
3. Arrange the mixed berries on top of the Greek yogurt.
4. Drizzle honey or maple syrup over the yogurt and berries for added sweetness, if desired.
5. Optional: Sprinkle granola on top for a delightful crunch and extra texture.
6. Garnish with fresh mint leaves for a burst of freshness and visual appeal.
7. Serve the Greek Yogurt with Berries immediately as a nutritious and delicious breakfast, snack, or dessert.

## Homemade Hummus with Veggie Sticks

**Ingredients:**
**For Homemade Hummus:**

- 1 can (15 oz) chickpeas, drained and rinsed
- 1/4 cup tahini
- 2 tablespoons lemon juice

- 2 cloves garlic, minced
- 1/2 teaspoon ground cumin
- 1/4 teaspoon paprika
- 1/4 cup olive oil
- Salt and black pepper to taste
- 2-3 tablespoons water (for adjusting consistency)

**For Veggie Sticks:**

- Carrot sticks
- Cucumber sticks
- Bell pepper strips (any color)

**Instructions:**

1. In a food processor, combine chickpeas, tahini, lemon juice, minced garlic, ground cumin, paprika, salt, and black pepper.
2. Pulse the ingredients until they are well blended and have a coarse texture.
3. While the food processor is running, slowly drizzle in the olive oil. Continue processing until the hummus becomes smooth and creamy.
4. If the hummus is too thick, add water, one tablespoon at a time, until you reach your desired consistency.

5. Taste the hummus and adjust the seasoning if needed.
6. Transfer the hummus to a serving bowl.
7. Wash and prepare the vegetable sticks (carrot, cucumber, and bell pepper).
8. Arrange the veggie sticks around the bowl of hummus for a colorful and appetizing presentation.
9. Optionally, drizzle a little olive oil over the hummus and sprinkle with a pinch of paprika.
10. Serve the Homemade Hummus with Veggie Sticks as a healthy and satisfying snack or appetizer.

## Trail Mix with Nuts and Dried Fruit

**Ingredients:**
- 1 cup almonds, raw or roasted
- 1 cup walnuts, raw or roasted
- 1 cup cashews, raw or roasted
- 1 cup dried cranberries
- 1 cup raisins
- 1/2 cup dark chocolate chips or chunks
- 1/2 cup pumpkin seeds (pepitas)
- 1/2 cup sunflower seeds

- 1/2 cup unsweetened coconut flakes
- Optional: 1/2 cup pretzels or whole grain cereal for added crunch

**Instructions:**

1. If using raw nuts, you can roast them for enhanced flavor. Preheat your oven to 350°F (175°C), spread the nuts on a baking sheet, and roast for about 8-10 minutes, stirring occasionally. Allow them to cool completely before proceeding.
2. In a large mixing bowl, combine the almonds, walnuts, cashews, dried cranberries, raisins, dark chocolate chips, pumpkin seeds, sunflower seeds, and coconut flakes.
3. If desired, break pretzels into smaller pieces and add them to the mix for an extra crunch.
4. Toss all the ingredients together until well combined.
5. Store the Trail Mix with Nuts and Dried Fruit in an airtight container or portion it into individual snack-sized bags for convenience.
6. Enjoy this homemade trail mix as a healthy and energy-boosting snack for hiking, work, or whenever you need a quick pick-me-up.

# Whole Grain Crackers with Avocado

**Ingredients:**

- Whole grain crackers (store-bought or homemade)
- 2 ripe avocados
- 1 tablespoon lemon juice
- Salt and black pepper to taste
- Optional toppings: cherry tomatoes, red pepper flakes, chives, or sesame seeds

**Instructions:**

1. In a bowl, scoop out the flesh of the ripe avocados.
2. Mash the avocados with a fork or potato masher until you achieve your desired level of smoothness.
3. Add lemon juice, salt, and black pepper to the mashed avocado. Mix well to combine.
4. Taste the avocado mixture and adjust the seasoning if needed.
5. Spread a generous amount of the avocado mixture onto each whole grain cracker.

6. Optional: Top the avocado-covered crackers with sliced cherry tomatoes, a sprinkle of red pepper flakes, chopped chives, or sesame seeds for added flavor and texture.
7. Arrange the avocado-topped crackers on a serving platter.
8. Serve the Whole Grain Crackers with Avocado as a quick and nutritious snack or appetizer.

## Cottage Cheese and Pineapple Cups

**Ingredients:**
- 1 cup cottage cheese
- 1 cup fresh pineapple, diced
- 2 tablespoons honey or maple syrup
- 1/4 cup shredded coconut
- 1/4 cup chopped nuts (such as almonds or walnuts)
- Mint leaves for garnish (optional)

**Instructions:**
1. In a bowl, mix together the cottage cheese and fresh pineapple.
2. Drizzle honey or maple syrup over the cottage cheese and pineapple mixture. Stir to combine.

3. In a dry skillet over medium heat, toast the shredded coconut and chopped nuts until they are golden brown and fragrant. This will take about 2-3 minutes. Be sure to stir frequently to prevent burning.
4. Sprinkle the toasted coconut and nuts over the cottage cheese and pineapple mixture. Gently fold them into the mixture.
5. Spoon the Cottage Cheese and Pineapple mixture into individual cups or bowls for serving.
6. Optionally, garnish each cup with fresh mint leaves for a burst of freshness.
7. Serve immediately as a refreshing and nutritious snack or breakfast.

## Baked Sweet Potato Fries

**Ingredients:**
- 2 large sweet potatoes, peeled and cut into fries
- 2 tablespoons olive oil
- 1 teaspoon paprika
- 1 teaspoon garlic powder
- 1 teaspoon onion powder
- 1/2 teaspoon cayenne pepper (adjust to taste)

- 1/2 teaspoon ground cumin
- Salt and black pepper to taste
- 2 tablespoons cornstarch (optional, for extra crispiness)

**Instructions:**

1. Preheat your oven to 425°F (220°C) and line a baking sheet with parchment paper.
2. In a large bowl, toss the sweet potato fries with olive oil until they are evenly coated.
3. In a small bowl, mix together paprika, garlic powder, onion powder, cayenne pepper, ground cumin, salt, and black pepper.
4. Sprinkle the spice mixture over the sweet potato fries, ensuring they are well coated. If you want extra crispiness, toss the fries with cornstarch at this point.
5. Spread the seasoned sweet potato fries in a single layer on the prepared baking sheet, ensuring they are not crowded to promote even baking.
6. Bake in the preheated oven for 20-25 minutes, flipping the fries halfway through, until they are golden brown and crispy.

7. Remove from the oven and let them cool for a few minutes before serving.
8. Serve the Baked Sweet Potato Fries with your favorite dipping sauce, such as ketchup, aioli, or yogurt-based dip.

## Edamame with Sea Salt

**Ingredients:**
- 2 cups frozen edamame in pods
- Sea salt (coarse or fine) for sprinkling

**Instructions:**
1. Bring a pot of water to a boil. Add a pinch of salt to the boiling water.
2. Add the frozen edamame pods to the boiling water. Cook for about 4-5 minutes or until they are tender.
3. Drain the edamame and transfer them to a bowl.
4. Sprinkle sea salt generously over the hot edamame while they are still moist. Toss them to coat evenly.
5. Allow the Edamame with Sea Salt to cool for a few minutes before serving.
6. Serve the edamame in a bowl, and provide an extra dish for discarded pods.

7. Optionally, sprinkle a bit more sea salt on top just before serving.
8. Enjoy these simple and nutritious Edamame with Sea Salt as a healthy snack or appetizer.

## Apple Slices with Almond Butter

**Ingredients:**
- 2 apples (any variety), cored and sliced
- 1/4 cup almond butter
- 1 tablespoon honey or maple syrup
- 1/2 teaspoon cinnamon (optional)
- 1/4 cup chopped almonds (optional, for extra crunch)
- Lemon juice (optional, to prevent browning of apples)

**Instructions:**
1. If you want to prevent the apple slices from browning, you can lightly toss them in lemon juice.
2. Arrange the apple slices on a serving plate or individual plates.
3. In a small bowl, mix almond butter, honey or maple syrup, and cinnamon until well combined.

4. Optionally, warm the almond butter mixture in the microwave for a few seconds to make it more drizzle-friendly.
5. Drizzle the almond butter mixture over the apple slices.
6. If desired, sprinkle chopped almonds over the top for added texture and crunch.
7. Serve the Apple Slices with Almond Butter immediately as a nutritious and satisfying snack.

## Kale Chips

**Ingredients:**

- 1 bunch of kale
- 1-2 tablespoons olive oil
- Salt, to taste
- Optional seasonings: garlic powder, onion powder, smoked paprika, nutritional yeast, or chili powder

**Instructions:**

1. Preheat your oven to 350°F (175°C).
2. Wash the kale leaves thoroughly and pat them dry with a kitchen towel. Remove the tough stems from the kale leaves.

3. Tear the kale leaves into bite-sized pieces, keeping in mind that they will shrink slightly during baking.
4. In a large bowl, drizzle olive oil over the kale leaves. Massage the oil into the leaves, ensuring they are well coated. You can use more or less oil depending on your preference.
5. Sprinkle salt over the kale leaves. Toss them to distribute the salt evenly.
6. Optionally, add your choice of seasonings such as garlic powder, onion powder, smoked paprika, nutritional yeast, or chili powder. Toss the leaves again to coat them evenly with the seasonings.
7. Line a baking sheet with parchment paper.
8. Arrange the seasoned kale leaves in a single layer on the prepared baking sheet. Avoid overcrowding to ensure even crisping.
9. Bake in the preheated oven for 10-15 minutes, checking after 10 minutes to prevent burning. The kale chips should be crisp but not browned.
10. Remove from the oven and let the kale chips cool on the baking sheet for a few minutes. They will continue to crisp up as they cool.

11. Transfer the Kale Chips to a serving bowl or enjoy them straight from the baking sheet.
12. Serve as a crunchy and nutritious snack.

## Chia Seed Pudding Cups

**Ingredients:**

- 1/4 cup chia seeds
- 1 cup almond milk (or any milk of your choice)
- 1-2 tablespoons maple syrup or honey (adjust to taste)
- 1/2 teaspoon vanilla extract
- Fresh berries, sliced fruits, or nuts for topping

**Instructions:**

1. In a bowl, combine chia seeds, almond milk, maple syrup or honey, and vanilla extract. Whisk the mixture thoroughly to ensure the chia seeds are well distributed.
2. Let the Chia Seed Pudding mixture sit for 5 minutes, and then whisk again to break up any clumps of chia seeds.
3. Cover the bowl and refrigerate the mixture for at least 3 hours, or preferably overnight. This allows the chia seeds to absorb the liquid and create a pudding-like consistency.

4. Before serving, give the Chia Seed Pudding a good stir to make sure it's well mixed.
5. Spoon the Chia Seed Pudding into individual cups or jars.
6. Top the pudding with fresh berries, sliced fruits, or nuts for added flavor and texture.
7. Optionally, drizzle a little extra maple syrup or honey on top for sweetness.
8. Serve the Chia Seed Pudding Cups chilled and enjoy this nutritious and customizable breakfast or snack.

## Roasted Chickpeas

**Ingredients:**
- 2 cans (15 oz each) chickpeas, drained and rinsed
- 2 tablespoons olive oil
- 1 teaspoon ground cumin
- 1 teaspoon smoked paprika
- 1/2 teaspoon garlic powder
- 1/2 teaspoon onion powder
- 1/4 teaspoon cayenne pepper (adjust to taste for spiciness)
- Salt and black pepper to taste

**Instructions:**
1. Preheat your oven to 400°F (200°C).
2. Rinse and drain the chickpeas. Pat them dry with a kitchen towel to remove excess moisture.
3. In a bowl, combine the chickpeas with olive oil, ground cumin, smoked paprika, garlic powder, onion powder, cayenne pepper, salt, and black pepper. Toss the chickpeas until they are evenly coated with the spice mixture.
4. Line a baking sheet with parchment paper or lightly grease it.
5. Spread the seasoned chickpeas in a single layer on the prepared baking sheet.
6. Bake in the preheated oven for 25-30 minutes, shaking the pan or stirring the chickpeas halfway through, until they are golden brown and crispy.
7. Remove from the oven and let the Roasted Chickpeas cool on the baking sheet. They will continue to crisp up as they cool.
8. Taste and adjust the seasoning if needed.
9. Serve the Roasted Chickpeas as a crunchy and flavorful snack or as a topping for salads, soups, or yogurt.

# Cucumber and Tuna Bites

**Ingredients:**

- 1 cucumber, cut into thick slices
- 1 can (5 oz) tuna, drained
- 2 tablespoons mayonnaise
- 1 tablespoon Dijon mustard
- 1 tablespoon fresh lemon juice
- Salt and black pepper to taste
- Cherry tomatoes, halved, for garnish
- Fresh parsley or dill, chopped, for garnish

**Instructions:**

1. In a bowl, combine drained tuna, mayonnaise, Dijon mustard, fresh lemon juice, salt, and black pepper. Mix well until all ingredients are evenly incorporated.
2. Place the cucumber slices on a serving platter or plate.
3. Spoon a small amount of the tuna mixture onto each cucumber slice.
4. Garnish each Cucumber and Tuna Bite with a halved cherry tomato.
5. Optionally, sprinkle chopped fresh parsley or dill over the bites for added flavor and visual appeal.

6. Serve immediately as a light and refreshing appetizer or snack.

## Cheese and Whole Grain Crackers

**Ingredients:**
- Assorted whole grain crackers
- 8 oz block of your favorite cheese (cheddar, gouda, Swiss, etc.)
- Grapes or apple slices for garnish (optional)
- Honey or fruit preserves for dipping (optional)

**Instructions:**
1. Arrange the whole grain crackers on a serving platter or board.
2. Using a sharp knife, cut the cheese into bite-sized cubes or thin slices.
3. Arrange the cheese pieces on the platter, ensuring they are evenly distributed among the crackers.
4. Optionally, add grapes or apple slices to the platter for a refreshing contrast.
5. Place a small bowl of honey or fruit preserves on the platter for dipping, if desired.
6. Serve the Cheese and Whole Grain Crackers as a delightful appetizer or snack.

# Fruit Smoothie

**Ingredients:**

- 1 cup frozen mixed berries (strawberries, blueberries, raspberries)
- 1 banana, peeled and sliced
- 1/2 cup plain Greek yogurt
- 1/2 cup orange juice
- 1/2 cup almond milk (or any milk of your choice)
- 1 tablespoon honey or maple syrup (optional, for sweetness)
- Ice cubes (optional, for a colder and thicker smoothie)

**Instructions:**

1. Place the frozen mixed berries, sliced banana, Greek yogurt, orange juice, almond milk, and honey or maple syrup (if using) in a blender.
2. If you prefer a thicker or colder smoothie, you can add a handful of ice cubes to the blender.
3. Blend the ingredients on high speed until the mixture is smooth and well combined. If the smoothie is too thick, you can add more almond milk or orange juice to reach your desired consistency.

4. Taste the smoothie and adjust the sweetness by adding more honey or maple syrup if needed.
5. Pour the Fruit Smoothie into glasses.
6. Optionally, garnish the smoothie with a few additional berries or a slice of banana for a decorative touch.
7. Serve the Fruit Smoothie immediately and enjoy as a refreshing and nutritious beverage.

## APPETIZERS

### Guacamole with Veggie Sticks

**Ingredients:**

**For Guacamole:**
- 3 ripe avocados, peeled and pitted
- 1 small red onion, finely diced
- 1-2 tomatoes, diced
- 1/4 cup fresh cilantro, chopped
- 1-2 cloves garlic, minced
- Juice of 1 lime
- Salt and black pepper to taste
- Optional: 1 jalapeño, seeded and finely chopped for heat

**For Veggie Sticks:**
- Carrot sticks
- Cucumber sticks
- Bell pepper strips (any color)

**Instructions:**
1. In a large mixing bowl, mash the ripe avocados with a fork or potato masher until you achieve your desired level of smoothness.
2. Add diced red onion, diced tomatoes, chopped cilantro, minced garlic, lime juice, salt, black pepper, and optional chopped jalapeño to the mashed avocados. Mix well to combine.
3. Taste the guacamole and adjust the seasoning or lime juice if needed.
4. Cover the bowl with plastic wrap, pressing it directly onto the surface of the guacamole to prevent browning. Refrigerate for at least 30 minutes to let the flavors meld.
5. Wash and prepare the vegetable sticks (carrot, cucumber, and bell pepper).
6. Arrange the guacamole in a serving bowl and surround it with the prepared veggie sticks.
7. Serve the Guacamole with Veggie Sticks as a flavorful and nutritious appetizer or snack.

## Quinoa-Stuffed Mushrooms

**Ingredients:**
- 12 large mushrooms, cleaned and stems removed
- 1 cup quinoa, rinsed
- 2 cups vegetable broth
- 1 tablespoon olive oil
- 1 small onion, finely chopped
- 2 cloves garlic, minced
- 1 cup spinach, chopped
- 1/2 cup cherry tomatoes, diced
- 1/4 cup feta cheese, crumbled
- 1/4 cup grated Parmesan cheese
- 1 teaspoon dried oregano
- 1 teaspoon dried thyme
- Salt and black pepper to taste
- Fresh parsley for garnish

**Instructions:**
1. Preheat your oven to 375°F (190°C).
2. In a medium saucepan, bring the vegetable broth to a boil. Add the rinsed quinoa, reduce the heat to low, cover, and simmer for about 15-20 minutes or until the quinoa is cooked and the liquid is absorbed.

3. While the quinoa is cooking, heat olive oil in a skillet over medium heat. Add chopped onion and sauté until it becomes translucent.
4. Add minced garlic to the skillet and stir for about 1 minute until fragrant.
5. Add chopped spinach to the skillet and cook until it wilts.
6. In a large mixing bowl, combine the cooked quinoa, sautéed onion, garlic, and spinach, diced cherry tomatoes, feta cheese, grated Parmesan, dried oregano, dried thyme, salt, and black pepper. Mix well to combine.
7. Clean the mushroom caps and remove the stems. Place the mushroom caps on a baking sheet.
8. Spoon the quinoa mixture into each mushroom cap, pressing it down gently.
9. Bake in the preheated oven for 20-25 minutes or until the mushrooms are tender and the stuffing is golden brown.
10. Remove from the oven and let the Quinoa-Stuffed Mushrooms cool for a few minutes.
11. Garnish with fresh parsley before serving.
12. Serve as an appetizer or a side dish.

# Smoked Salmon Cucumber Bites

**Ingredients:**

- 1 English cucumber, cut into thick slices
- 4 oz smoked salmon, thinly sliced
- 1/4 cup cream cheese
- 1 tablespoon fresh dill, chopped
- 1 teaspoon capers (optional, for garnish)
- Lemon wedges for serving

**Instructions:**

1. Slice the cucumber into thick rounds, creating a base for the Smoked Salmon Cucumber Bites.
2. In a small bowl, mix the cream cheese with chopped fresh dill until well combined.
3. Spread a small amount of the dill-infused cream cheese onto each cucumber slice.
4. Carefully drape a slice of smoked salmon over the cream cheese on each cucumber round.
5. Garnish each bite with capers, if desired.
6. Arrange the Smoked Salmon Cucumber Bites on a serving platter.
7. Serve with lemon wedges on the side for squeezing over the bites.
8. Enjoy these elegant and flavorful bites as an appetizer or snack.

# Greek Yogurt and Herb Dip

**Ingredients:**

- 1 cup Greek yogurt (full-fat or low-fat)
- 2 tablespoons fresh parsley, finely chopped
- 1 tablespoon fresh dill, finely chopped
- 1 tablespoon fresh chives, finely chopped
- 1 clove garlic, minced
- 1 tablespoon lemon juice
- 1 tablespoon extra-virgin olive oil
- Salt and black pepper to taste

**Instructions:**

1. In a bowl, combine Greek yogurt, finely chopped parsley, dill, chives, minced garlic, lemon juice, and extra-virgin olive oil.
2. Mix the ingredients thoroughly to ensure an even distribution of herbs and flavors.
3. Season the Greek Yogurt and Herb Dip with salt and black pepper to taste. Adjust the seasoning according to your preference.
4. Cover the bowl with plastic wrap and refrigerate the dip for at least 30 minutes to allow the flavors to meld.
5. Before serving, give the dip a final stir.

6. Transfer the Greek Yogurt and Herb Dip to a serving bowl.
7. Optionally, garnish the dip with additional chopped herbs or a drizzle of olive oil.
8. Serve the dip with vegetable sticks, pita chips, or as a refreshing accompaniment to various dishes.

## Caprese Skewers

**Ingredients:**

- Cherry tomatoes
- Fresh mozzarella balls (bocconcini)
- Fresh basil leaves
- Balsamic glaze or balsamic reduction
- Extra-virgin olive oil
- Salt and black pepper to taste
- Toothpicks or small skewers

**Instructions:**

1. Rinse the cherry tomatoes and pat them dry with a paper towel.
2. Drain the fresh mozzarella balls if they are stored in liquid.
3. Assemble the Caprese Skewers by threading a cherry tomato onto a toothpick or skewer, followed by a fresh basil leaf, and then a mozzarella ball.

4. Repeat the process until you have as many skewers as desired.
5. Arrange the Caprese Skewers on a serving platter.
6. In a small bowl, whisk together balsamic glaze or reduction, extra-virgin olive oil, salt, and black pepper. Adjust the ingredients to taste.
7. Drizzle the balsamic glaze mixture over the Caprese Skewers just before serving.
8. Optionally, sprinkle a bit of extra salt and pepper on top.
9. Serve the Caprese Skewers immediately as a refreshing and flavorful appetizer.

## Roasted Red Pepper Hummus

**Ingredients:**

- 1 can (15 oz) chickpeas, drained and rinsed
- 1/2 cup roasted red peppers (from a jar or homemade)
- 1/4 cup tahini
- 2 tablespoons lemon juice
- 2 cloves garlic, minced
- 1/2 teaspoon ground cumin
- 1/4 teaspoon cayenne pepper (optional, for heat)

- Salt and black pepper to taste
- 1/4 cup extra-virgin olive oil
- Water (as needed for consistency)

**Instructions:**

1. In a food processor, combine chickpeas, roasted red peppers, tahini, lemon juice, minced garlic, ground cumin, cayenne pepper (if using), salt, and black pepper.
2. Pulse the ingredients until they are well blended and have a smooth consistency.
3. While the food processor is running, slowly drizzle in the extra-virgin olive oil. Continue processing until the hummus becomes creamy.
4. If the hummus is too thick, you can add water, one tablespoon at a time, until you reach your desired consistency.
5. Taste the Roasted Red Pepper Hummus and adjust the seasoning if needed.
6. Transfer the hummus to a serving bowl.
7. Optionally, drizzle a little extra-virgin olive oil on top and garnish with a sprinkle of cayenne pepper or chopped fresh parsley.

8. Serve the Roasted Red Pepper Hummus with pita bread, vegetable sticks, or as a spread on sandwiches.

## Spinach and Artichoke Dip

**Ingredients:**

- 1 cup frozen chopped spinach, thawed and drained
- 1 can (14 oz) artichoke hearts, drained and chopped
- 1/2 cup mayonnaise
- 1/2 cup sour cream
- 1 cup shredded mozzarella cheese
- 1/2 cup grated Parmesan cheese
- 1 teaspoon garlic powder
- Salt and black pepper to taste
- 1/4 teaspoon red pepper flakes (optional, for heat)
- 1 tablespoon olive oil (for greasing baking dish)
- Tortilla chips, pita chips, or sliced baguette for serving

**Instructions:**

1. Preheat your oven to 375°F (190°C).

2. In a mixing bowl, combine chopped spinach, chopped artichoke hearts, mayonnaise, sour cream, shredded mozzarella, grated Parmesan, garlic powder, salt, black pepper, and red pepper flakes if using.
3. Mix the ingredients until well combined.
4. Lightly grease a baking dish with olive oil.
5. Transfer the spinach and artichoke mixture into the prepared baking dish, spreading it evenly.
6. Bake in the preheated oven for about 25-30 minutes or until the dip is hot and bubbly, and the top is golden brown.
7. Remove from the oven and let the Spinach and Artichoke Dip cool for a few minutes before serving.
8. Serve the dip with tortilla chips, pita chips, or sliced baguette.

## Sautéed Shrimp with Garlic and Lemon

**Ingredients:**

- 1 pound large shrimp, peeled and deveined
- 3 tablespoons olive oil
- 4 cloves garlic, minced

- 1 teaspoon red pepper flakes (adjust to taste, for heat)
- Salt and black pepper to taste
- Zest of 1 lemon
- Juice of 1 lemon
- 2 tablespoons fresh parsley, chopped

**Instructions:**

1. Pat the shrimp dry with a paper towel and season them with salt and black pepper.
2. In a large skillet or pan, heat olive oil over medium-high heat.
3. Add minced garlic and red pepper flakes to the hot oil, sautéing for about 1-2 minutes until the garlic becomes fragrant. Be careful not to burn the garlic.
4. Add the seasoned shrimp to the skillet in a single layer. Cook for 2-3 minutes on one side until they start to turn pink.
5. Flip the shrimp to cook the other side, and continue cooking for an additional 2-3 minutes until the shrimp are opaque and fully cooked.
6. Add lemon zest and lemon juice to the skillet, tossing the shrimp to coat them evenly with the lemony goodness.

7. Taste the Sautéed Shrimp with Garlic and Lemon and adjust the seasoning if needed.
8. Sprinkle chopped fresh parsley over the shrimp and toss one last time.
9. Remove the skillet from the heat.
10. Serve the Sautéed Shrimp with Garlic and Lemon immediately over rice, pasta, or with crusty bread.

## Vegetable Spring Rolls

**Ingredients:**

**For the Spring Rolls:**
- Rice paper wrappers
- 1 cup vermicelli rice noodles, cooked according to package instructions
- 1 cup shredded carrots
- 1 cucumber, julienned
- 1 bell pepper, thinly sliced
- 1 cup purple cabbage, thinly sliced
- Fresh mint leaves
- Fresh cilantro leaves
- Cooked and peeled shrimp or tofu (optional)
- Sesame seeds (optional, for garnish)

**For the Dipping Sauce:**
- 1/4 cup soy sauce
- 2 tablespoons hoisin sauce
- 1 tablespoon rice vinegar
- 1 teaspoon sesame oil
- 1 teaspoon honey or maple syrup (optional)
- 1 clove garlic, minced
- 1/2 teaspoon grated ginger
- Red pepper flakes (optional, for heat)

**Instructions:**
1. Prepare all the vegetables and set them aside.
2. If using shrimp, cook and peel them. If using tofu, cut it into thin strips.
3. Cook the vermicelli rice noodles according to the package instructions. Drain and set aside.
4. Fill a large shallow bowl with warm water. Dip one rice paper wrapper into the water for about 5-10 seconds until it becomes pliable.
5. Place the wet rice paper on a clean, damp surface, such as a cutting board.
6. In the center of the rice paper, layer a small amount of vermicelli rice noodles, shredded carrots, julienned cucumber, sliced bell pepper, purple cabbage, fresh mint leaves, cilantro leaves, and optional shrimp or tofu.

7. Fold the sides of the rice paper inward, then tightly roll the wrapper from the bottom to the top, creating a neat spring roll.
8. Repeat the process with the remaining rice paper wrappers and fillings.
9. Arrange the Vegetable Spring Rolls on a serving platter.
10. In a small bowl, whisk together soy sauce, hoisin sauce, rice vinegar, sesame oil, honey or maple syrup (if using), minced garlic, grated ginger, and red pepper flakes (if using). Adjust the flavors according to your preference.
11. Optionally, sprinkle sesame seeds over the Vegetable Spring Rolls for garnish.
12. Serve the spring rolls with the dipping sauce on the side.

## Egg White Deviled Eggs

**Ingredients:**

- 6 large hard-boiled eggs, cooled and peeled
- 3/4 cup egg whites (from the hard-boiled eggs)
- 2 tablespoons non-fat Greek yogurt
- 1 tablespoon Dijon mustard
- 1 teaspoon white vinegar

- Salt and black pepper to taste
- Paprika for garnish
- Fresh chives or parsley for garnish (optional)

**Instructions:**

1. Cut the hard-boiled eggs in half lengthwise. Carefully remove the yolks and place them in a bowl. Set the egg whites aside.
2. To the bowl with egg yolks, add egg whites, non-fat Greek yogurt, Dijon mustard, white vinegar, salt, and black pepper.
3. Mash and mix the ingredients together until you achieve a smooth and creamy consistency.
4. Taste the egg white mixture and adjust the seasoning if needed.
5. Spoon the egg white mixture into a piping bag or a plastic sandwich bag with one corner snipped off.
6. Pipe the egg white mixture into the hollowed egg whites, creating a mound on top.
7. Optionally, sprinkle a pinch of paprika over each Egg White Deviled Egg for color and flavor.
8. Garnish with fresh chives or parsley if desired.
9. Arrange the Egg White Deviled Eggs on a serving platter.

10. Chill in the refrigerator for at least 30 minutes before serving.
11. Serve these healthier Deviled Eggs as a light and protein-packed appetizer or snack.

## Avocado and Tomato Bruschetta

**Ingredients:**
- Baguette or Italian bread, sliced
- 2 ripe avocados, peeled and diced
- 1 cup cherry tomatoes, diced
- 1/4 cup red onion, finely chopped
- 2 tablespoons fresh basil, chopped
- 1 clove garlic, minced
- 2 tablespoons extra-virgin olive oil
- 1 tablespoon balsamic vinegar
- Salt and black pepper to taste
- Optional: Balsamic glaze for drizzling

**Instructions:**
1. Preheat your oven broiler or grill.
2. Place the bread slices on a baking sheet and toast them under the broiler or on the grill for 1-2 minutes on each side until they are golden brown.

3. In a bowl, combine diced avocados, diced cherry tomatoes, chopped red onion, chopped basil, minced garlic, extra-virgin olive oil, balsamic vinegar, salt, and black pepper.
4. Mix the ingredients gently until well combined. Taste and adjust the seasoning if needed.
5. Allow the Avocado and Tomato Bruschetta mixture to sit for a few minutes to let the flavors meld.
6. Spoon the bruschetta mixture onto the toasted bread slices.
7. Optionally, drizzle a bit of balsamic glaze over the top for extra flavor.
8. Arrange the Avocado and Tomato Bruschetta on a serving platter.
9. Serve immediately as a tasty and refreshing appetizer.

## Cucumber Cups with Tuna Salad

**Ingredients:**

- 2 large cucumbers
- 1 can (5 oz) tuna, drained
- 1/4 cup mayonnaise
- 1 tablespoon Dijon mustard

- 2 tablespoons red onion, finely chopped
- 2 tablespoons celery, finely chopped
- 1 tablespoon fresh dill, chopped
- Salt and black pepper to taste
- Cherry tomatoes for garnish (optional)

**Instructions:**

1. Peel the cucumbers, leaving alternating strips of skin for a decorative effect. Cut the cucumbers into thick slices, about 1.5 inches each.
2. Use a melon baller or a small spoon to scoop out the seeds from the center of each cucumber slice, creating a small cup. Be careful not to scoop too deep, leaving a sturdy base for the cups.
3. In a bowl, combine drained tuna, mayonnaise, Dijon mustard, chopped red onion, chopped celery, chopped fresh dill, salt, and black pepper. Mix well until all ingredients are evenly incorporated.
4. Taste the tuna salad and adjust the seasoning if needed.
5. Spoon the tuna salad into each cucumber cup, creating a mound on top.
6. Optionally, garnish each Cucumber Cup with Tuna Salad with a halved cherry tomato for a colorful touch.
7. Arrange the cucumber cups on a serving platter.

8. Serve immediately as a light and refreshing appetizer or snack.

## Zucchini Fritters

**Ingredients:**
- 2 medium zucchinis, grated
- 1 teaspoon salt
- 1/2 cup all-purpose flour
- 1/4 cup grated Parmesan cheese
- 2 cloves garlic, minced
- 1/4 cup fresh parsley, chopped
- 2 large eggs, beaten
- 1/4 teaspoon black pepper
- Olive oil for frying
- Greek yogurt or sour cream for serving (optional)

**Instructions:**
1. Place the grated zucchini in a colander over the sink and sprinkle it with salt. Let it sit for about 10 minutes to allow excess water to drain.
2. After 10 minutes, use your hands or a clean kitchen towel to squeeze out the excess moisture from the grated zucchini.

3. In a large bowl, combine the grated zucchini, all-purpose flour, grated Parmesan cheese, minced garlic, chopped fresh parsley, beaten eggs, and black pepper. Mix well until all ingredients are evenly incorporated.
4. Heat a few tablespoons of olive oil in a large skillet over medium heat.
5. Spoon portions of the zucchini mixture into the skillet, flattening them slightly to form fritters. Cook for 3-4 minutes on each side or until they are golden brown and crispy.
6. Remove the Zucchini Fritters from the skillet and place them on a plate lined with paper towels to absorb any excess oil.
7. Repeat the process until all the zucchini mixture is used, adding more olive oil to the skillet as needed.
8. Serve the Zucchini Fritters warm with a side of Greek yogurt or sour cream for dipping, if desired.

# CHAPTER 7: SALADS AND DESSERTS

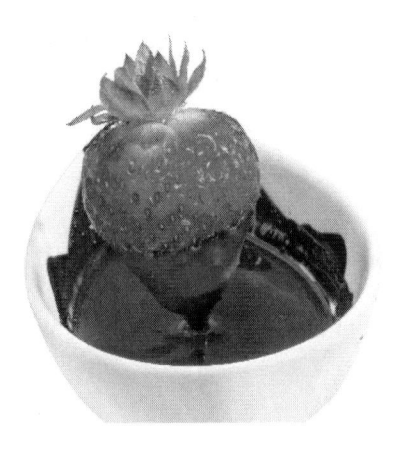

## SALADS

### Kale and Berry Salad

**Ingredients:**

**For the Salad:**

- 6 cups kale, stems removed and leaves chopped
- 1 cup strawberries, hulled and sliced
- 1/2 cup blueberries
- 1/2 cup blackberries
- 1/4 cup toasted almond slices
- 1/4 cup crumbled feta cheese (optional)

**For the Dressing:**
- 3 tablespoons extra-virgin olive oil
- 2 tablespoons balsamic vinegar
- 1 tablespoon honey
- 1 teaspoon Dijon mustard
- Salt and black pepper to taste

**Instructions:**
1. In a large salad bowl, combine chopped kale, sliced strawberries, blueberries, blackberries, toasted almond slices, and crumbled feta cheese (if using).
2. In a small bowl, whisk together extra-virgin olive oil, balsamic vinegar, honey, Dijon mustard, salt, and black pepper to create the dressing.
3. Pour the dressing over the kale and berry mixture.
4. Toss the salad well to ensure all ingredients are evenly coated with the dressing.
5. Let the Kale and Berry Salad sit for a few minutes to allow the flavors to meld.
6. Serve the salad immediately as a refreshing and nutritious side dish.

## Quinoa and Chickpea Salad

**Ingredients:**

**For the Salad:**

- 1 cup quinoa, rinsed
- 2 cups water or vegetable broth
- 1 can (15 oz) chickpeas, drained and rinsed
- 1 cucumber, diced
- 1 red bell pepper, diced
- 1/2 red onion, finely chopped
- 1 cup cherry tomatoes, halved
- 1/4 cup Kalamata olives, sliced
- 1/4 cup fresh parsley, chopped
- Feta cheese, crumbled (optional)

**For the Dressing:**

- 1/4 cup extra-virgin olive oil
- 2 tablespoons red wine vinegar
- 1 teaspoon Dijon mustard
- 1 clove garlic, minced
- 1/2 teaspoon dried oregano
- Salt and black pepper to taste

**Instructions:**

1. In a medium saucepan, combine quinoa and water or vegetable broth.

2. Bring to a boil, then reduce the heat to low, cover, and simmer for 15-20 minutes or until the quinoa is cooked and the liquid is absorbed. Fluff the quinoa with a fork and let it cool.
3. In a large salad bowl, combine cooked quinoa, drained chickpeas, diced cucumber, diced red bell pepper, chopped red onion, halved cherry tomatoes, sliced Kalamata olives, and chopped fresh parsley.
4. In a small bowl, whisk together extra-virgin olive oil, red wine vinegar, Dijon mustard, minced garlic, dried oregano, salt, and black pepper to create the dressing.
5. Pour the dressing over the quinoa and chickpea mixture.
6. Toss the salad gently until all ingredients are well coated with the dressing.
7. Optionally, sprinkle crumbled feta cheese over the top.
8. Let the Quinoa and Chickpea Salad sit for a few minutes to allow the flavors to meld.
9. Serve the salad chilled or at room temperature as a wholesome and satisfying meal.

# Spinach and Pomegranate Salad

**Ingredients:**

**For the Salad:**

- 6 cups fresh baby spinach
- 1 cup pomegranate arils (seeds)
- 1/2 cup crumbled feta cheese
- 1/2 cup sliced almonds, toasted
- 1 medium red onion, thinly sliced

**For the Dressing:**

- 1/4 cup extra-virgin olive oil
- 2 tablespoons balsamic vinegar
- 1 tablespoon honey
- 1 teaspoon Dijon mustard
- Salt and black pepper to taste

**Instructions:**

1. In a large salad bowl, combine fresh baby spinach, pomegranate arils, crumbled feta cheese, toasted sliced almonds, and thinly sliced red onion.
2. In a small bowl, whisk together extra-virgin olive oil, balsamic vinegar, honey, Dijon mustard, salt, and black pepper to create the dressing.

3. Pour the dressing over the spinach and pomegranate mixture.
4. Toss the salad gently until all ingredients are well coated with the dressing.
5. Let the Spinach and Pomegranate Salad sit for a few minutes to allow the flavors to meld.
6. Serve the salad immediately as a vibrant and nutritious side dish.

## Grilled Chicken and Avocado Salad

**Ingredients:**

**For the Grilled Chicken:**
- 2 boneless, skinless chicken breasts
- 2 tablespoons olive oil
- 1 teaspoon paprika
- 1 teaspoon garlic powder
- 1 teaspoon dried thyme
- Salt and black pepper to taste

**For the Salad:**
- 6 cups mixed salad greens (lettuce, spinach, arugula, etc.)
- 1 cucumber, sliced
- 1 cup cherry tomatoes, halved
- 1 avocado, sliced

- 1/4 cup red onion, thinly sliced
- 1/4 cup feta cheese, crumbled

**For the Dressing:**
- 1/4 cup extra-virgin olive oil
- 2 tablespoons balsamic vinegar
- 1 teaspoon Dijon mustard
- 1 clove garlic, minced
- Salt and black pepper to taste

**Instructions:**
1. Preheat the grill to medium-high heat.
2. In a bowl, mix olive oil, paprika, garlic powder, dried thyme, salt, and black pepper. Coat the chicken breasts with this mixture.
3. Grill the chicken breasts for about 6-8 minutes per side or until they are cooked through and have nice grill marks. Ensure the internal temperature reaches 165°F (74°C).
4. Remove the grilled chicken from the grill and let it rest for a few minutes before slicing it into strips.
5. In a large salad bowl, combine mixed salad greens, sliced cucumber, halved cherry tomatoes, sliced avocado, thinly sliced red onion, and crumbled feta cheese.

6. In a small bowl, whisk together extra-virgin olive oil, balsamic vinegar, Dijon mustard, minced garlic, salt, and black pepper to create the dressing.
7. Pour the dressing over the salad ingredients.
8. Toss the salad gently until all ingredients are well coated with the dressing.
9. Top the salad with the sliced grilled chicken.
10. Serve the Grilled Chicken and Avocado Salad immediately as a delicious and satisfying main course.

## Cabbage and Apple Slaw

**Ingredients:**

**For the Slaw:**

- 4 cups shredded green cabbage
- 2 cups shredded red cabbage
- 2 apples, cored and julienned
- 1 cup shredded carrots
- 1/2 cup chopped fresh parsley

**For the Dressing:**

- 1/3 cup mayonnaise
- 2 tablespoons Dijon mustard
- 2 tablespoons apple cider vinegar

- 1 tablespoon honey
- Salt and black pepper to taste

**Optional Add-ins:**
- 1/2 cup raisins or dried cranberries
- 1/4 cup chopped walnuts or pecans

**Instructions:**
1. In a large bowl, combine shredded green cabbage, shredded red cabbage, julienned apples, shredded carrots, and chopped fresh parsley.
2. In a separate small bowl, whisk together mayonnaise, Dijon mustard, apple cider vinegar, honey, salt, and black pepper to create the dressing.
3. Pour the dressing over the cabbage and apple mixture.
4. Toss the slaw gently until all ingredients are well coated with the dressing.
5. If desired, add raisins or dried cranberries and chopped nuts (walnuts or pecans) to the slaw and toss again.
6. Let the Cabbage and Apple Slaw sit in the refrigerator for at least 30 minutes before serving to allow the flavors to meld.

7. Serve the slaw chilled as a refreshing and crunchy side dish.

## Mango and Black Bean Salad

**Ingredients:**

**For the Salad:**

- 2 ripe mangoes, peeled, pitted, and diced
- 1 can (15 oz) black beans, drained and rinsed
- 1 red bell pepper, diced
- 1/2 red onion, finely chopped
- 1 cup cherry tomatoes, halved
- 1/4 cup fresh cilantro, chopped

**For the Dressing:**

- 3 tablespoons lime juice
- 2 tablespoons extra-virgin olive oil
- 1 tablespoon honey
- 1 teaspoon ground cumin
- 1/2 teaspoon chili powder
- Salt and black pepper to taste

**Instructions:**

1. In a large bowl, combine diced mangoes, drained black beans, diced red bell pepper, finely chopped red onion, halved cherry tomatoes, and chopped fresh cilantro.

2. In a small bowl, whisk together lime juice, extra-virgin olive oil, honey, ground cumin, chili powder, salt, and black pepper to create the dressing.
3. Pour the dressing over the mango and black bean mixture.
4. Toss the salad gently until all ingredients are well coated with the dressing.
5. Let the Mango and Black Bean Salad sit in the refrigerator for at least 15-20 minutes before serving to allow the flavors to meld.
6. Serve the salad chilled as a flavorful and refreshing side dish.

## Tuna and White Bean Salad

**Ingredients:**

**For the Salad:**

- 2 cans (15 oz each) white beans (cannellini or great northern), drained and rinsed
- 2 cans (5 oz each) tuna in water, drained
- 1/2 red onion, finely chopped
- 1/2 cup cherry tomatoes, halved
- 1/4 cup Kalamata olives, sliced
- 1/4 cup fresh parsley, chopped

**For the Dressing:**
- 1/4 cup extra-virgin olive oil
- 2 tablespoons red wine vinegar
- 1 teaspoon Dijon mustard
- 1 clove garlic, minced
- Salt and black pepper to taste

**Instructions:**
1. In a large bowl, combine drained and rinsed white beans, drained tuna, finely chopped red onion, halved cherry tomatoes, sliced Kalamata olives, and chopped fresh parsley.
2. In a small bowl, whisk together extra-virgin olive oil, red wine vinegar, Dijon mustard, minced garlic, salt, and black pepper to create the dressing.
3. Pour the dressing over the tuna and white bean mixture.
4. Toss the salad gently until all ingredients are well coated with the dressing.
5. Let the Tuna and White Bean Salad sit in the refrigerator for at least 15-20 minutes before serving to allow the flavors to meld.
6. Serve the salad chilled as a protein-packed and flavorful main course or side dish.

# Roasted Vegetable Quinoa Salad

**Ingredients:**

**For the Salad:**

- 1 cup quinoa, rinsed
- 2 cups water or vegetable broth
- 1 cup cherry tomatoes, halved
- 1 zucchini, diced
- 1 red bell pepper, diced
- 1 yellow bell pepper, diced
- 1 small red onion, thinly sliced
- 1 cup broccoli florets
- 2 tablespoons olive oil
- Salt and black pepper to taste
- 1/4 cup crumbled feta cheese (optional)
- Fresh basil or parsley for garnish

**For the Dressing:**

- 1/4 cup extra-virgin olive oil
- 2 tablespoons balsamic vinegar
- 1 clove garlic, minced
- 1 teaspoon Dijon mustard
- Salt and black pepper to taste

**Instructions:**

1. Preheat the oven to 425°F (220°C).

2. In a saucepan, combine quinoa and water or vegetable broth. Bring to a boil, then reduce the heat to low, cover, and simmer for 15-20 minutes or until the quinoa is cooked and the liquid is absorbed. Fluff with a fork and let it cool.
3. In a large mixing bowl, combine halved cherry tomatoes, diced zucchini, diced red and yellow bell peppers, thinly sliced red onion, and broccoli florets.
4. Drizzle olive oil over the vegetables, and season with salt and black pepper. Toss the vegetables until they are evenly coated.
5. Spread the vegetables on a baking sheet in a single layer.
6. Roast the vegetables in the preheated oven for about 20-25 minutes or until they are tender and slightly caramelized, stirring once or twice during roasting.
7. In a small bowl, whisk together extra-virgin olive oil, balsamic vinegar, minced garlic, Dijon mustard, salt, and black pepper to create the dressing.

8. In a large salad bowl, combine cooked quinoa, roasted vegetables, and crumbled feta cheese if using.
9. Pour the dressing over the salad and toss gently to combine.
10. Garnish with fresh basil or parsley.
11. Serve the Roasted Vegetable Quinoa Salad at room temperature or chilled.

## Broccoli and Walnut Salad

**Ingredients:**

**For the Salad:**
- 4 cups broccoli florets, blanched
- 1/2 cup chopped walnuts, toasted
- 1/2 cup red grapes, halved
- 1/4 cup red onion, finely chopped
- 1/4 cup crumbled feta cheese (optional)
- 2 tablespoons fresh parsley, chopped

**For the Dressing:**
- 1/4 cup mayonnaise
- 2 tablespoons Greek yogurt
- 1 tablespoon apple cider vinegar
- 1 tablespoon honey
- Salt and black pepper to taste

**Instructions:**

1. Blanch the broccoli florets in boiling water for about 2 minutes, then immediately transfer them to an ice bath to stop the cooking process. Drain and pat them dry.
2. In a dry skillet, toast the chopped walnuts over medium heat for 2-3 minutes or until they become fragrant. Be careful not to burn them.
3. In a large salad bowl, combine blanched broccoli florets, toasted walnuts, halved red grapes, finely chopped red onion, crumbled feta cheese (if using), and chopped fresh parsley.
4. In a small bowl, whisk together mayonnaise, Greek yogurt, apple cider vinegar, honey, salt, and black pepper to create the dressing.
5. Pour the dressing over the broccoli and walnut mixture.
6. Toss the salad gently until all ingredients are well coated with the dressing.
7. Let the Broccoli and Walnut Salad sit in the refrigerator for at least 30 minutes before serving to allow the flavors to meld.
8. Serve the salad chilled as a crisp and flavorful side dish.

# Caprese Salad with Whole Grain Croutons

**Ingredients:**

**For the Salad:**

- 4 large tomatoes, sliced
- 8 ounces fresh mozzarella cheese, sliced
- Fresh basil leaves
- Balsamic glaze for drizzling
- Salt and black pepper to taste

**For the Whole Grain Croutons:**

- 2 cups whole grain bread, cut into cubes
- 2 tablespoons olive oil
- 1 teaspoon dried Italian herbs (basil, oregano, thyme)
- Salt and black pepper to taste

**Instructions:**

1. Preheat the oven to 375°F (190°C).
2. In a bowl, toss the whole grain bread cubes with olive oil, dried Italian herbs, salt, and black pepper until the cubes are evenly coated.
3. Spread the seasoned bread cubes on a baking sheet in a single layer.

4. Bake the whole grain croutons in the preheated oven for about 10-15 minutes or until they are golden brown and crisp, stirring occasionally to ensure even toasting.
5. Remove the croutons from the oven and let them cool.
6. On a serving platter, arrange sliced tomatoes, fresh mozzarella cheese, and fresh basil leaves in an alternating pattern.
7. Sprinkle the whole grain croutons over the Caprese Salad.
8. Drizzle balsamic glaze over the salad for added flavor.
9. Season the Caprese Salad with salt and black pepper to taste.
10. Serve the salad immediately as a light and refreshing appetizer or side dish.

## Cucumber and Feta Greek Salad

**Ingredients:**

**For the Salad:**

- 4 medium cucumbers, diced
- 1 cup cherry tomatoes, halved
- 1/2 red onion, thinly sliced

- 1 cup Kalamata olives, pitted and sliced
- 1 cup crumbled feta cheese
- Fresh dill or oregano for garnish (optional)

**For the Dressing:**
- 1/4 cup extra-virgin olive oil
- 2 tablespoons red wine vinegar
- 1 teaspoon dried oregano
- 1 clove garlic, minced
- Salt and black pepper to taste

**Instructions:**
1. In a large salad bowl, combine diced cucumbers, halved cherry tomatoes, thinly sliced red onion, sliced Kalamata olives, and crumbled feta cheese.
2. In a small bowl, whisk together extra-virgin olive oil, red wine vinegar, dried oregano, minced garlic, salt, and black pepper to create the dressing.
3. Pour the dressing over the cucumber and feta mixture.
4. Toss the salad gently until all ingredients are well coated with the dressing.

5. Let the Cucumber and Feta Greek Salad sit in the refrigerator for at least 15-20 minutes before serving to allow the flavors to meld.
6. Optionally, garnish the salad with fresh dill or oregano.
7. Serve the salad chilled as a refreshing and tangy side dish.

## Sweet Potato and Kale Salad

**Ingredients:**

**For the Salad:**

- 2 large sweet potatoes, peeled and diced
- 1 bunch kale, stems removed and leaves chopped
- 1/2 cup dried cranberries
- 1/2 cup pecans, chopped and toasted
- 1/4 cup red onion, thinly sliced
- Feta or goat cheese, crumbled (optional)

**For the Dressing:**

- 1/4 cup olive oil
- 2 tablespoons apple cider vinegar
- 1 tablespoon maple syrup
- 1 teaspoon Dijon mustard
- Salt and black pepper to taste

**Instructions:**
1. Preheat the oven to 400°F (200°C).
2. Toss the diced sweet potatoes with a bit of olive oil, salt, and black pepper. Spread them on a baking sheet in a single layer and roast for about 20-25 minutes or until they are tender and golden, stirring halfway through.
3. In a large salad bowl, combine chopped kale, dried cranberries, toasted pecans, and thinly sliced red onion.
4. Once the sweet potatoes are roasted, let them cool for a few minutes, then add them to the salad.
5. In a small bowl, whisk together olive oil, apple cider vinegar, maple syrup, Dijon mustard, salt, and black pepper to create the dressing.
6. Pour the dressing over the salad and toss gently until all ingredients are well coated.
7. If desired, sprinkle crumbled feta or goat cheese over the top for added creaminess.
8. Let the Sweet Potato and Kale Salad sit for a few minutes to allow the flavors to meld.
9. Serve the salad at room temperature or chilled as a hearty and flavorful side dish.

# DESSERTS

## Berry and Yogurt Parfait

**Ingredients:**

- 2 cups Greek yogurt (plain or vanilla)
- 1 cup granola
- 1 cup mixed berries (strawberries, blueberries, raspberries)
- Honey for drizzling (optional)
- Mint leaves for garnish (optional)

**Instructions:**

1. In serving glasses or bowls, start by layering a spoonful of Greek yogurt at the bottom.
2. Add a layer of granola on top of the yogurt.
3. Place a portion of mixed berries over the granola.
4. Repeat the layers until the glass or bowl is filled, ending with a layer of berries on top.
5. Drizzle honey over the parfait for added sweetness if desired.
6. Garnish with fresh mint leaves for a burst of freshness.
7. Serve the Berry and Yogurt Parfait immediately as a delightful and healthy breakfast or dessert.

# Dark Chocolate-Dipped Strawberries

**Ingredients:**

- 1 pound fresh strawberries, washed and dried
- 8 ounces dark chocolate (70% cocoa or higher), chopped
- 1 tablespoon coconut oil (optional, for smoother consistency)
- Toppings (optional): chopped nuts, shredded coconut, sprinkles

**Instructions:**

1. Line a baking sheet with parchment paper.
2. In a heatproof bowl, melt the dark chocolate using a double boiler or in the microwave in 20-second intervals, stirring between each interval. If using, add coconut oil to the chocolate for a smoother consistency.
3. Hold each strawberry by the stem and dip it into the melted chocolate, swirling to coat it evenly. Allow any excess chocolate to drip back into the bowl.
4. Place the chocolate-dipped strawberries on the prepared baking sheet.

5. If desired, immediately sprinkle toppings like chopped nuts, shredded coconut, or sprinkles over the chocolate before it sets.
6. Allow the chocolate to set at room temperature or speed up the process by placing the baking sheet in the refrigerator for about 15-20 minutes.
7. Once the chocolate is completely set, transfer the dark chocolate-dipped strawberries to a serving plate or box.
8. Serve the Dark Chocolate-Dipped Strawberries as a decadent and elegant dessert.

## Chia Seed Chocolate Pudding

**Ingredients:**
- 1/4 cup chia seeds
- 1 cup unsweetened almond milk (or any milk of your choice)
- 2 tablespoons cocoa powder
- 2-3 tablespoons maple syrup or honey (adjust to taste)
- 1/2 teaspoon vanilla extract
- A pinch of salt
- Fresh berries or sliced fruits for topping (optional)

**Instructions:**

1. In a bowl, whisk together chia seeds, unsweetened almond milk, cocoa powder, maple syrup (or honey), vanilla extract, and a pinch of salt.
2. Continue to whisk the mixture for a couple of minutes to ensure that the chia seeds are well distributed and don't clump together.
3. Cover the bowl and refrigerate the Chia Seed Chocolate Pudding for at least 3 hours or overnight. Stir the mixture once or twice during the first hour to prevent clumping.
4. After the pudding has set and thickened, give it a good stir to break up any lumps.
5. Serve the Chia Seed Chocolate Pudding in individual bowls or jars.
6. Optionally, top the pudding with fresh berries or sliced fruits.
7. Enjoy this delicious and healthy Chia Seed Chocolate Pudding as a satisfying dessert or breakfast treat!

# Baked Apples with Cinnamon

**Ingredients:**

- 4 large apples (such as Honeycrisp or Granny Smith)
- 1/4 cup brown sugar
- 1 teaspoon ground cinnamon
- 1/4 teaspoon ground nutmeg
- 1 tablespoon unsalted butter, diced
- 1/2 cup water or apple juice
- Vanilla ice cream or whipped cream for serving (optional)

**Instructions:**

1. Preheat the oven to 375°F (190°C).
2. Wash and core the apples, leaving the bottoms intact to form a well for the filling.
3. In a small bowl, mix together brown sugar, ground cinnamon, and ground nutmeg.
4. Place the cored apples in a baking dish.
5. Stuff each apple with the brown sugar and cinnamon mixture, dividing it evenly among the apples.
6. Place a small piece of diced butter on top of each stuffed apple.

7. Pour water or apple juice into the bottom of the baking dish.
8. Bake the apples in the preheated oven for about 30-40 minutes or until they are tender but not mushy. Baking time may vary depending on the size and type of apples.
9. Optionally, baste the apples with the liquid from the bottom of the baking dish during baking to keep them moist.
10. Remove the baked apples from the oven and let them cool slightly before serving.
11. Serve the Baked Apples with Cinnamon warm, optionally topped with vanilla ice cream or whipped cream.

## Avocado Chocolate Mousse

**Ingredients:**
- 2 ripe avocados, peeled and pitted
- 1/4 cup unsweetened cocoa powder
- 1/4 cup maple syrup or agave nectar
- 1/4 cup almond milk (or any milk of your choice)
- 1 teaspoon vanilla extract
- A pinch of salt

- Optional toppings: shaved chocolate, berries, chopped nuts

**Instructions:**
1. In a food processor or blender, combine the ripe avocados, unsweetened cocoa powder, maple syrup (or agave nectar), almond milk, vanilla extract, and a pinch of salt.
2. Blend the ingredients until the mixture is smooth and creamy, scraping down the sides of the blender or food processor as needed.
3. Taste the Avocado Chocolate Mousse and adjust the sweetness if necessary by adding more maple syrup or agave nectar.
4. Once the mixture is smooth and well combined, transfer the chocolate mousse to serving glasses or bowls.
5. Refrigerate the Avocado Chocolate Mousse for at least 1-2 hours to chill and allow the flavors to meld.
6. Before serving, optionally garnish the mousse with shaved chocolate, berries, or chopped nuts.
7. Serve the Avocado Chocolate Mousse chilled as a rich and indulgent dessert.

## Frozen Banana Bites

**Ingredients:**

- 2 ripe bananas
- 1/4 cup peanut butter or almond butter
- 1/2 cup dark chocolate chips or melting chocolate
- Toppings of your choice (chopped nuts, shredded coconut, sprinkles)

**Instructions:**

1. Peel the ripe bananas and cut them into bite-sized slices, about 1/2 inch thick.
2. Spread a small amount of peanut butter or almond butter on half of the banana slices.
3. Create banana "sandwiches" by placing the remaining banana slices on top of the ones spread with nut butter.
4. Insert toothpicks into the center of each banana "sandwich" to create bite-sized pops.
5. Place the banana bites on a parchment paper-lined tray and freeze for at least 1-2 hours or until they are firm.
6. In a microwave-safe bowl, melt the dark chocolate chips in 20-second intervals, stirring between each interval until smooth. Alternatively, you can melt the chocolate using a double boiler.

7. Remove the frozen banana bites from the freezer.
8. Dip each banana bite into the melted chocolate, coating them evenly.
9. Allow any excess chocolate to drip off before placing the banana bites back on the parchment paper.
10. Quickly sprinkle your choice of toppings over the chocolate-covered banana bites before the chocolate sets.
11. Return the tray to the freezer and freeze the banana bites for an additional 1-2 hours or until the chocolate is fully set.
12. Once frozen, remove the toothpicks and serve the Frozen Banana Bites as a delicious and refreshing frozen treat.

## Coconut and Berry Sorbet

**Ingredients:**

- 2 cups mixed berries (strawberries, blueberries, raspberries)
- 1 can (13.5 oz) coconut milk (full fat)
- 1/3 cup honey or maple syrup (adjust to taste)
- 1 teaspoon vanilla extract

- Pinch of salt
- Unsweetened shredded coconut for garnish (optional)

**Instructions:**
1. In a blender, combine mixed berries, coconut milk, honey or maple syrup, vanilla extract, and a pinch of salt.
2. Blend the ingredients until you achieve a smooth and well-combined mixture.
3. Taste the sorbet mixture and adjust the sweetness if needed by adding more honey or maple syrup.
4. Pour the sorbet mixture into an ice cream maker and churn according to the manufacturer's instructions until it reaches a soft-serve consistency.
5. If you don't have an ice cream maker, you can pour the mixture into a shallow dish and freeze it. Every 30 minutes, stir the mixture with a fork to break up ice crystals until it reaches the desired sorbet consistency.
6. Once the sorbet has reached the desired consistency, transfer it to a lidded container and freeze for an additional 2-3 hours to firm up.

7. Before serving, let the Coconut and Berry Sorbet sit at room temperature for a few minutes to soften slightly.
8. Optionally, garnish the sorbet with unsweetened shredded coconut before serving.
9. Scoop the sorbet into bowls or cones and enjoy this dairy-free and refreshing treat.

## Date and Nut Energy Balls

**Ingredients:**

- 1 cup Medjool dates, pitted
- 1 cup nuts (such as almonds, walnuts, or a mix), unsalted
- 1/4 cup shredded coconut (unsweetened)
- 1 tablespoon chia seeds (optional)
- 1 tablespoon flaxseeds (optional)
- 1 teaspoon vanilla extract
- A pinch of salt
- Additional shredded coconut or crushed nuts for rolling (optional)

**Instructions:**
1. In a food processor, combine pitted Medjool dates, nuts, shredded coconut, chia seeds (if using), flaxseeds (if using), vanilla extract, and a pinch of salt.
2. Pulse the mixture until it forms a sticky and crumbly consistency. Stop and scrape down the sides of the food processor as needed.
3. Test the mixture by pressing a small amount between your fingers. If it holds together, it's ready. If not, pulse a bit more.
4. Take about a tablespoon of the mixture and roll it between your palms to form a ball. If the mixture is too sticky, you can wet your hands with water.
5. If desired, roll the energy balls in additional shredded coconut or crushed nuts for extra texture.
6. Repeat the rolling process until all the mixture is used.
7. Place the Date and Nut Energy Balls on a parchment paper-lined tray or plate.
8. Refrigerate the energy balls for at least 30 minutes to firm up.

9. Once chilled, transfer the energy balls to an airtight container and store them in the refrigerator for longer freshness.
10. Enjoy these Date and Nut Energy Balls as a quick and nutritious snack.

## Baked Peaches with Almonds

**Ingredients:**
- 4 ripe peaches, halved and pitted
- 2 tablespoons unsalted butter, melted
- 2 tablespoons honey or maple syrup
- 1 teaspoon vanilla extract
- 1/2 teaspoon ground cinnamon
- 1/4 cup sliced almonds
- Greek yogurt or vanilla ice cream for serving (optional)

**Instructions:**
1. Preheat the oven to 375°F (190°C).
2. Place the halved and pitted peaches in a baking dish, cut side up.
3. In a small bowl, mix melted butter, honey or maple syrup, vanilla extract, and ground cinnamon.

4. Brush the honey-butter mixture over the cut sides of the peaches, ensuring they are well coated.
5. Sprinkle sliced almonds over the top of each peach half.
6. Bake the peaches in the preheated oven for about 20-25 minutes or until they are tender and the almonds are golden brown.
7. Remove the baked peaches from the oven and let them cool slightly.
8. Serve the Baked Peaches with Almonds warm, optionally with a dollop of Greek yogurt or a scoop of vanilla ice cream.
9. Drizzle any remaining honey-butter mixture from the baking dish over the top before serving.

## Pumpkin Pie Smoothie

**Ingredients:**
- 1/2 cup canned pumpkin puree
- 1/2 large banana, frozen
- 1 cup unsweetened almond milk (or any milk of your choice)
- 1/2 cup Greek yogurt (plain or vanilla)

- 1 tablespoon maple syrup or honey (adjust to taste)
- 1/2 teaspoon pumpkin pie spice (or a mix of cinnamon, nutmeg, and cloves)
- 1/2 teaspoon vanilla extract
- Ice cubes (optional)

**Instructions:**

1. In a blender, combine canned pumpkin puree, frozen banana, almond milk, Greek yogurt, maple syrup or honey, pumpkin pie spice, and vanilla extract.
2. If you prefer a colder smoothie, you can add a handful of ice cubes to the blender.
3. Blend the ingredients until smooth and creamy. If needed, stop and scrape down the sides of the blender to ensure everything is well combined.
4. Taste the Pumpkin Pie Smoothie and adjust the sweetness or spice levels to your liking.
5. Pour the smoothie into a glass.
6. Optionally, sprinkle a bit of additional pumpkin pie spice on top for garnish.
7. Serve the Pumpkin Pie Smoothie immediately as a festive and flavorful treat.

# Cinnamon-Spiced Roasted Pears

**Ingredients:**

- 4 ripe but firm pears, halved and cored
- 2 tablespoons unsalted butter, melted
- 3 tablespoons honey or maple syrup
- 1 teaspoon ground cinnamon
- 1/4 teaspoon ground nutmeg
- A pinch of salt
- Chopped nuts (such as walnuts or pecans) for garnish (optional)
- Greek yogurt or vanilla ice cream for serving (optional)

**Instructions:**

1. Preheat the oven to 375°F (190°C).
2. Place the halved and cored pears in a baking dish, cut side up.
3. In a small bowl, mix melted butter, honey or maple syrup, ground cinnamon, ground nutmeg, and a pinch of salt.
4. Brush the cinnamon-spiced mixture over the cut sides of the pears, ensuring they are well coated.
5. Roast the pears in the preheated oven for about 25-30 minutes or until they are tender and slightly caramelized.

6. While roasting, baste the pears with the juices from the baking dish a couple of times to keep them moist.
7. Remove the roasted pears from the oven and let them cool slightly.
8. Optionally, sprinkle chopped nuts over the top for added texture and flavor.
9. Serve the Cinnamon-Spiced Roasted Pears warm, optionally with a dollop of Greek yogurt or a scoop of vanilla ice cream.
10. Drizzle any remaining cinnamon-spiced mixture from the baking dish over the top before serving.

## Yogurt and Berry Popsicles

**Ingredients:**
- 2 cups Greek yogurt (plain or vanilla)
- 1 cup mixed berries (strawberries, blueberries, raspberries)
- 2-3 tablespoons honey or maple syrup (adjust to taste)
- 1 teaspoon vanilla extract
- Popsicle molds
- Popsicle sticks

**Instructions:**

1. In a bowl, mix Greek yogurt, mixed berries, honey or maple syrup, and vanilla extract until well combined.
2. Taste the mixture and adjust the sweetness if needed by adding more honey or maple syrup.
3. Spoon the yogurt and berry mixture into popsicle molds, layering it evenly.
4. Tap the molds on the counter to remove air bubbles and ensure the mixture settles evenly.
5. Insert popsicle sticks into the molds, making sure they are centered.
6. Freeze the Yogurt and Berry Popsicles for at least 4-6 hours, or until completely frozen.
7. Once frozen, run the molds briefly under warm water to loosen the popsicles.
8. Carefully remove the popsicles from the molds.
9. Serve the Yogurt and Berry Popsicles immediately for a refreshing and healthy frozen treat.

## Oatmeal Raisin Cookies

**Ingredients:**

- 1 cup unsalted butter, softened

- 1 cup brown sugar, packed
- 1/2 cup granulated sugar
- 2 large eggs
- 1 teaspoon vanilla extract
- 1 1/2 cups all-purpose flour
- 1 teaspoon baking soda
- 1 teaspoon ground cinnamon
- 1/2 teaspoon salt
- 3 cups old-fashioned rolled oats
- 1 cup raisins

**Instructions:**

1. Preheat the oven to 350°F (175°C). Line baking sheets with parchment paper.
2. In a large bowl, cream together softened butter, brown sugar, and granulated sugar until light and fluffy.
3. Add eggs one at a time, beating well after each addition. Stir in vanilla extract.
4. In a separate bowl, whisk together flour, baking soda, ground cinnamon, and salt.
5. Gradually add the dry ingredients to the wet ingredients, mixing until just combined.
6. Stir in old-fashioned rolled oats and raisins until evenly distributed in the cookie dough.

7. Drop rounded tablespoons of cookie dough onto the prepared baking sheets, spacing them about 2 inches apart.
8. Bake in the preheated oven for 10-12 minutes or until the edges are golden brown but the centers are still soft.
9. Allow the Oatmeal Raisin Cookies to cool on the baking sheets for 5 minutes before transferring them to wire racks to cool completely.
10. Store the cooled cookies in an airtight container at room temperature.

"With each wholesome bite, I am nourishing both body and spirit."

"I trust in the healing properties of the foods I include in my diet."

# CHAPTER 8: HERBS AND SPICES

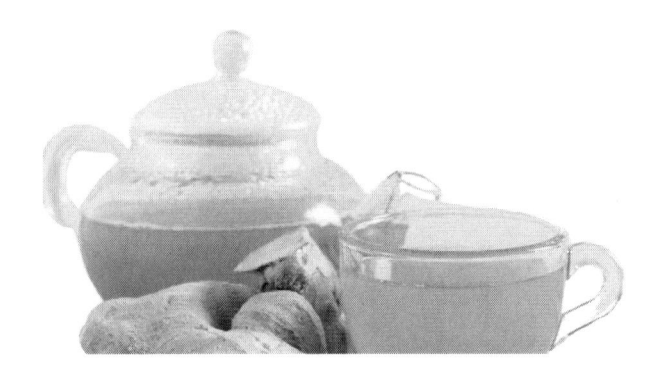

## Turmeric-Ginger Tea

**Ingredients:**

- 2 cups water
- 1 teaspoon turmeric powder (or 1 tablespoon grated fresh turmeric)
- 1 teaspoon ginger, grated
- 1-2 teaspoons honey (adjust to taste)
- 1/2 lemon, juiced (optional)
- Pinch of black pepper (enhances turmeric absorption)
- Fresh mint leaves for garnish (optional)

**Instructions:**
1. In a small saucepan, bring 2 cups of water to a simmer.
2. Add turmeric powder (or grated fresh turmeric) and grated ginger to the simmering water.
3. Allow the mixture to simmer for about 5-10 minutes, stirring occasionally.
4. Remove the saucepan from heat and let the turmeric-ginger mixture steep for an additional 5 minutes.
5. Strain the tea into a cup to remove the turmeric and ginger particles.
6. Stir in honey to sweeten the tea, adjusting the amount to your taste preference.
7. Optionally, add freshly squeezed lemon juice for added brightness.
8. Add a pinch of black pepper to enhance the absorption of turmeric's beneficial compounds.
9. Garnish the Turmeric-Ginger Tea with fresh mint leaves if desired.
10. Stir well and serve the tea hot.

# Garlic and Herb Roasted Vegetables

**Ingredients:**

- 4 cups mixed vegetables (such as carrots, potatoes, bell peppers, zucchini, and cherry tomatoes), washed and chopped
- 3 tablespoons olive oil
- 4 cloves garlic, minced
- 1 teaspoon dried thyme
- 1 teaspoon dried rosemary
- 1 teaspoon dried oregano
- Salt and black pepper to taste
- Fresh parsley for garnish (optional)

**Instructions:**

1. Preheat the oven to 425°F (220°C). Line a baking sheet with parchment paper.
2. In a large bowl, combine the mixed vegetables with olive oil, minced garlic, dried thyme, dried rosemary, dried oregano, salt, and black pepper. Toss until the vegetables are evenly coated with the seasonings.
3. Spread the seasoned vegetables in a single layer on the prepared baking sheet.

4. Roast the Garlic and Herb Roasted Vegetables in the preheated oven for 25-30 minutes or until they are tender and golden brown, stirring halfway through the cooking time.
5. Remove the baking sheet from the oven and let the roasted vegetables cool slightly.
6. Garnish the vegetables with fresh parsley if desired.
7. Serve the Garlic and Herb Roasted Vegetables as a flavorful and nutritious side dish.

## Basil Pesto Sauce

**Ingredients:**
- 2 cups fresh basil leaves, packed
- 1/2 cup freshly grated Parmesan cheese
- 1/2 cup pine nuts or walnuts
- 3 garlic cloves, peeled
- 1 cup extra-virgin olive oil
- Salt and black pepper to taste
- 1/2 cup freshly grated Pecorino Romano cheese (optional)

**Instructions:**
1. In a food processor, combine fresh basil leaves, grated Parmesan cheese, pine nuts or walnuts, and peeled garlic cloves.
2. Pulse the ingredients until coarsely chopped.
3. With the food processor running, gradually add the extra-virgin olive oil in a steady stream. Continue processing until the mixture becomes a smooth paste.
4. Stop the food processor and scrape down the sides to ensure all ingredients are well incorporated.
5. Season the Basil Pesto Sauce with salt and black pepper to taste. Pulse briefly to combine.
6. If desired, add freshly grated Pecorino Romano cheese and pulse again until just combined.
7. Taste the pesto and adjust the salt and pepper as needed.
8. Transfer the Basil Pesto Sauce to a jar or airtight container.
9. Store the pesto in the refrigerator for immediate use or cover the surface with a thin layer of olive oil to prevent oxidation and freezer for later use.

# Cilantro-Lime Quinoa

**Ingredients:**

- 1 cup quinoa, rinsed and drained
- 2 cups vegetable or chicken broth (or water)
- 1 bunch fresh cilantro, chopped
- 1-2 limes, juiced
- 2 tablespoons olive oil
- 2 cloves garlic, minced
- Salt and black pepper to taste

**Instructions:**

1. In a medium saucepan, combine quinoa and vegetable or chicken broth (or water). Bring to a boil over medium-high heat.
2. Reduce the heat to low, cover, and simmer for 15-20 minutes, or until the quinoa is cooked and the liquid is absorbed.
3. While the quinoa is cooking, prepare the dressing. In a small bowl, whisk together lime juice, olive oil, minced garlic, salt, and black pepper.
4. Once the quinoa is cooked, fluff it with a fork and transfer it to a large bowl.
5. Pour the cilantro-lime dressing over the quinoa and toss to combine.

6. Add chopped fresh cilantro to the quinoa and mix well.
7. Taste the Cilantro-Lime Quinoa and adjust the seasoning if needed by adding more salt, pepper, or lime juice.
8. Serve the quinoa warm as a side dish or as a base for protein and vegetable bowls.

## Mint-Infused Fruit Salad

**Ingredients:**
- 2 cups fresh pineapple chunks
- 2 cups fresh watermelon cubes
- 1 cup fresh strawberries, hulled and halved
- 1 cup green grapes, halved
- 1 cup blueberries
- 1/4 cup fresh mint leaves, chopped
- 2 tablespoons honey or maple syrup (optional)
- Juice of 1 lime or lemon

**Instructions:**
1. In a large bowl, combine fresh pineapple chunks, watermelon cubes, halved strawberries, halved green grapes, and blueberries.

2. In a small bowl, mix chopped fresh mint leaves with honey or maple syrup (if using) and lime or lemon juice.
3. Pour the mint-infused dressing over the fruit salad.
4. Gently toss the fruit salad to coat it evenly with the mint-infused dressing.
5. Let the Mint-Infused Fruit Salad sit in the refrigerator for at least 30 minutes to allow the flavors to meld.
6. Before serving, toss the fruit salad once more and garnish with additional fresh mint leaves if desired.
7. Serve the Mint-Infused Fruit Salad as a refreshing and vibrant side dish or dessert.

## Rosemary Lemon Grilled Chicken

**Ingredients:**

- 4 boneless, skinless chicken breasts
- 1/4 cup olive oil
- 2 tablespoons fresh rosemary, chopped
- Zest of 1 lemon
- Juice of 1 lemon
- 3 cloves garlic, minced

- Salt and black pepper to taste
- Lemon slices and fresh rosemary sprigs for garnish

**Instructions:**

1. In a bowl, whisk together olive oil, chopped fresh rosemary, lemon zest, lemon juice, minced garlic, salt, and black pepper to create the marinade.
2. Place the chicken breasts in a resealable plastic bag or a shallow dish.
3. Pour the rosemary lemon marinade over the chicken, ensuring each piece is well coated. Seal the bag or cover the dish and refrigerate for at least 30 minutes to marinate.
4. Preheat the grill to medium-high heat.
5. Remove the chicken from the refrigerator and let it come to room temperature for about 10 minutes.
6. Grease the grill grates to prevent sticking.
7. Grill the Rosemary Lemon Grilled Chicken for approximately 6-8 minutes per side, or until the internal temperature reaches 165°F (74°C) and the chicken is cooked through.

8. During the last few minutes of grilling, baste the chicken with any remaining marinade for added flavor.
9. Remove the chicken from the grill and let it rest for a few minutes before serving.
10. Garnish the Rosemary Lemon Grilled Chicken with lemon slices and fresh rosemary sprigs.
11. Serve the grilled chicken with your favorite side dishes.

## Chia Seed Cinnamon Pudding

**Ingredients:**

- 1/4 cup chia seeds
- 1 cup almond milk (or any milk of your choice)
- 1-2 tablespoons maple syrup or honey (adjust to taste)
- 1/2 teaspoon ground cinnamon
- 1/2 teaspoon vanilla extract
- A pinch of salt
- Fresh berries or sliced fruits for topping (optional)

**Instructions:**

1. In a bowl, combine chia seeds, almond milk, maple syrup or honey, ground cinnamon, vanilla extract, and a pinch of salt.
2. Whisk the mixture until well combined.
3. Cover the bowl and refrigerate the Chia Seed Cinnamon Pudding for at least 3 hours or overnight. Stir the mixture once or twice during the first hour to prevent clumping.
4. After the pudding has set and thickened, give it a good stir to break up any lumps.
5. Taste the Chia Seed Cinnamon Pudding and adjust the sweetness if necessary by adding more maple syrup or honey.
6. Once the mixture is smooth and well combined, transfer the pudding to serving glasses or bowls.
7. Optionally, top the pudding with fresh berries or sliced fruits.
8. Serve the Chia Seed Cinnamon Pudding chilled as a satisfying dessert or breakfast treat.

## Thyme and Lemon Baked Salmon

**Ingredients:**

- 4 salmon filets

- 2 tablespoons olive oil
- 2 tablespoons fresh thyme leaves
- Zest of 1 lemon
- Juice of 1 lemon
- 2 cloves garlic, minced
- Salt and black pepper to taste
- Lemon slices for garnish
- Fresh thyme sprigs for garnish

**Instructions:**

1. Preheat the oven to 375°F (190°C). Line a baking sheet with parchment paper.
2. Place the salmon filets on the prepared baking sheet.
3. In a small bowl, whisk together olive oil, fresh thyme leaves, lemon zest, lemon juice, minced garlic, salt, and black pepper to create the marinade.
4. Pour the thyme and lemon marinade over the salmon filets, ensuring each piece is well coated. You can also use a brush to spread the marinade evenly.
5. Let the salmon marinate for at least 15-20 minutes to allow the flavors to infuse.

6. Bake the Thyme and Lemon Baked Salmon in the preheated oven for about 15-20 minutes or until the salmon is cooked through and flakes easily with a fork.
7. During baking, you can baste the salmon with the marinade a couple of times for added flavor.
8. Remove the salmon from the oven and let it rest for a few minutes.
9. Garnish the Thyme and Lemon Baked Salmon with lemon slices and fresh thyme sprigs.
10. Serve the baked salmon with your favorite side dishes.

## Coriander-Cumin Roasted Chickpeas

**Ingredients:**
- 2 cans (15 ounces each) chickpeas, drained and rinsed
- 2 tablespoons olive oil
- 1 teaspoon ground coriander
- 1 teaspoon ground cumin
- 1/2 teaspoon smoked paprika
- 1/2 teaspoon garlic powder
- 1/4 teaspoon cayenne pepper (adjust to taste)
- Salt to taste

- Freshly ground black pepper to taste
- 1 tablespoon chopped fresh cilantro (optional, for garnish)

**Instructions:**
1. Preheat your oven to 400°F (200°C).
2. Rinse and drain the chickpeas thoroughly. Pat them dry with a paper towel to remove excess moisture.
3. In a bowl, combine the chickpeas, olive oil, ground coriander, ground cumin, smoked paprika, garlic powder, cayenne pepper, salt, and black pepper. Mix well, ensuring that the chickpeas are evenly coated with the spices.
4. Spread the seasoned chickpeas in a single layer on a baking sheet lined with parchment paper. This ensures even roasting.
5. Bake in the preheated oven for about 25-30 minutes or until the chickpeas are golden brown and crispy. Shake the baking sheet or stir the chickpeas halfway through the baking time for even crispiness.
6. Remove the chickpeas from the oven and let them cool for a few minutes.

7. If desired, sprinkle chopped fresh cilantro over the roasted chickpeas for a burst of freshness.
8. Serve the coriander-cumin roasted chickpeas as a snack or a crunchy topping for salads. Enjoy!

## Dill Yogurt Sauce

**Ingredients:**
- 1 cup plain Greek yogurt
- 2 tablespoons fresh dill, finely chopped
- 1 tablespoon lemon juice
- 1 clove garlic, minced
- 1/2 teaspoon Dijon mustard
- Salt and pepper to taste

**Instructions:**
1. In a bowl, combine the plain Greek yogurt, finely chopped fresh dill, lemon juice, minced garlic, and Dijon mustard.
2. Mix the ingredients thoroughly to ensure an even distribution of flavors.
3. Taste the mixture and add salt and pepper according to your preference. Stir again to incorporate the seasoning.

4. Cover the bowl with plastic wrap or a lid and refrigerate the dill yogurt sauce for at least 30 minutes before serving. This allows the flavors to meld and intensify.
5. Before serving, give the sauce a final stir to make sure the ingredients are well combined.
6. Use the dill yogurt sauce as a refreshing dip for vegetables, a topping for grilled meats, or a flavorful dressing for salads.

## Oregano and Tomato Quinoa Salad

**Ingredients:**
- 1 cup quinoa, rinsed and drained
- 2 cups water or vegetable broth
- 1 cup cherry tomatoes, halved
- 1/2 cup cucumber, diced
- 1/4 cup red onion, finely chopped
- 1/4 cup Kalamata olives, sliced
- 1/4 cup feta cheese, crumbled (optional)
- 2 tablespoons fresh oregano, chopped
- 3 tablespoons extra-virgin olive oil
- 2 tablespoons red wine vinegar
- Salt and pepper to taste

**Instructions:**
1. In a medium saucepan, combine the quinoa and water or vegetable broth. Bring to a boil, then reduce heat to low, cover, and simmer for 15-20 minutes or until the quinoa is cooked and the liquid is absorbed. Fluff the quinoa with a fork and let it cool to room temperature.
2. In a large mixing bowl, combine the cooked quinoa, cherry tomatoes, cucumber, red onion, Kalamata olives, and feta cheese (if using).
3. In a small bowl, whisk together the extra-virgin olive oil, red wine vinegar, chopped fresh oregano, salt, and pepper to create the dressing.
4. Pour the dressing over the quinoa mixture and toss gently to coat all the ingredients evenly.
5. Taste the salad and adjust the seasoning if needed.
6. Allow the oregano and tomato quinoa salad to chill in the refrigerator for at least 30 minutes to let the flavors meld.
7. Before serving, give the salad a gentle stir and garnish with additional fresh oregano if desired.
8. Serve the quinoa salad as a refreshing side dish or a light, nutritious main course.

# Sage and Butternut Squash Soup

**Ingredients:**

- 1 medium-sized butternut squash, peeled, seeded, and diced
- 1 onion, chopped
- 2 carrots, peeled and chopped
- 2 celery stalks, chopped
- 2 cloves garlic, minced
- 4 cups vegetable or chicken broth
- 2 tablespoons olive oil
- 1 teaspoon dried sage
- 1/2 teaspoon ground nutmeg
- Salt and pepper to taste
- 1 cup coconut milk or heavy cream (optional, for added creaminess)
- Fresh sage leaves for garnish (optional)

**Instructions:**

1. In a large pot, heat the olive oil over medium heat. Add the chopped onion, carrots, celery, and garlic. Sauté until the vegetables are softened, about 5-7 minutes.
2. Add the diced butternut squash to the pot and continue to sauté for an additional 5 minutes.

3. Pour in the vegetable or chicken broth, ensuring that the vegetables are well covered. Bring the mixture to a boil, then reduce the heat to low, cover, and simmer until the butternut squash is tender, about 20-25 minutes.
4. Once the vegetables are soft, use an immersion blender to puree the soup until smooth. Alternatively, transfer the soup to a blender in batches, being cautious with hot liquids.
5. Stir in the dried sage, ground nutmeg, salt, and pepper. Adjust the seasonings to taste.
6. If you desire extra creaminess, add coconut milk or heavy cream to the soup and stir until well combined. Adjust the consistency by adding more broth if needed.
7. Simmer the soup for an additional 5-10 minutes to allow the flavors to meld.
8. Ladle the sage and butternut squash soup into bowls and garnish with fresh sage leaves if desired.
9. Serve the soup hot, accompanied by crusty bread or croutons.

# Paprika-Spiced Sweet Potato Wedges

**Ingredients:**

- 2 large sweet potatoes, washed and scrubbed
- 2 tablespoons olive oil
- 1 teaspoon smoked paprika
- 1/2 teaspoon sweet paprika
- 1/2 teaspoon garlic powder
- 1/2 teaspoon onion powder
- 1/2 teaspoon dried thyme
- 1/2 teaspoon salt
- 1/4 teaspoon black pepper

**Instructions:**

1. Preheat your oven to 425°F (220°C) and line a baking sheet with parchment paper.
2. Cut the sweet potatoes into wedges by halving them lengthwise and then cutting each half into wedges.
3. In a large bowl, combine the olive oil, smoked paprika, sweet paprika, garlic powder, onion powder, dried thyme, salt, and black pepper. Mix well to create a spice blend.
4. Add the sweet potato wedges to the bowl and toss them in the spice blend until evenly coated.

5. Arrange the seasoned sweet potato wedges in a single layer on the prepared baking sheet, ensuring they are not crowded to promote even cooking and crispiness.
6. Bake in the preheated oven for 25-30 minutes, turning the wedges halfway through the baking time to ensure they cook evenly.
7. Check for doneness by inserting a fork into a wedge; they should be tender inside and crispy on the outside.
8. Once the paprika-spiced sweet potato wedges are cooked to perfection, remove them from the oven and let them cool for a few minutes before serving.
9. Optionally, garnish with fresh herbs like chopped parsley or chives.
10. Serve the sweet potato wedges as a delicious and flavorful side dish or snack.

## Chamomile Lavender Smoothie

**Ingredients:**

- 1 cup chamomile tea, cooled (brewed and chilled)
- 1 banana, peeled and frozen

- 1/2 cup plain Greek yogurt
- 1/2 cup frozen blueberries
- 1 tablespoon honey (adjust to taste)
- 1/2 teaspoon dried lavender buds (culinary-grade)
- Ice cubes (optional)

**Instructions:**

1. Brew chamomile tea and allow it to cool. Once cooled, refrigerate it until cold or use ice cubes to speed up the chilling process.
2. In a blender, combine the cooled chamomile tea, frozen banana, plain Greek yogurt, frozen blueberries, honey, and dried lavender buds.
3. Blend on high speed until all the ingredients are well combined and the smoothie reaches your desired consistency.
4. Taste the smoothie and adjust sweetness by adding more honey if needed.
5. If you prefer a colder smoothie, you can add a handful of ice cubes and blend again until smooth.
6. Pour the chamomile lavender smoothie into glasses.

7. Optionally, garnish with a sprinkle of dried lavender buds for a decorative touch.
8. Serve the smoothie immediately and enjoy the calming and aromatic flavors.

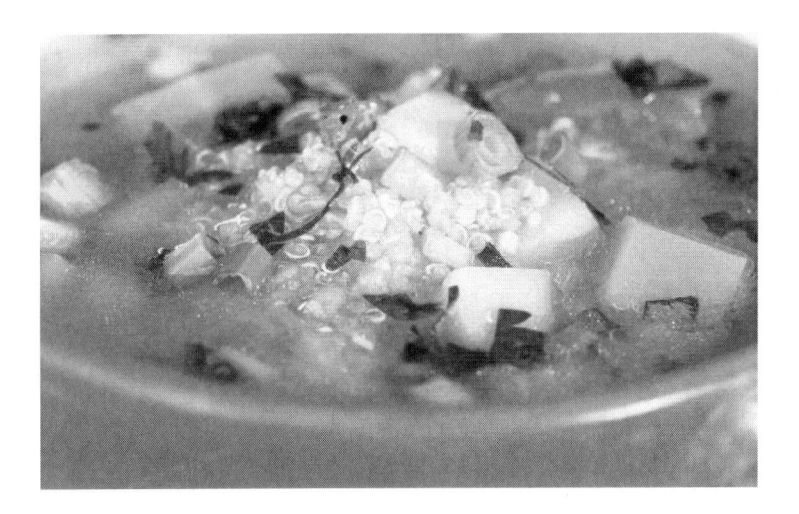

"I am on a journey of wellness, and my diet supports my vibrant life."

"Every nutrient I consume contributes to my overall health and vitality."

# CHAPTER 9: SOUPS AND STEWS

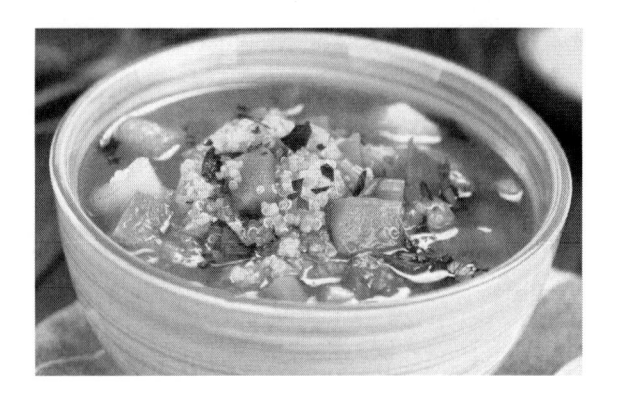

## SOUPS

### Anti-Inflammatory Turmeric Soup

**Ingredients:**

- 1 tablespoon olive oil
- 1 onion, finely chopped
- 2 carrots, peeled and diced
- 2 celery stalks, diced
- 3 cloves garlic, minced
- 1 tablespoon fresh ginger, grated
- 1 teaspoon ground turmeric
- 1/2 teaspoon ground cumin
- 1/2 teaspoon ground coriander
- 1/4 teaspoon cayenne pepper (adjust to taste)

- 1 cup red lentils, rinsed and drained
- 6 cups vegetable broth
- 1 can (14 ounces) diced tomatoes
- 1 cup kale, stems removed and leaves chopped
- Juice of 1 lemon
- Salt and pepper to taste
- Fresh cilantro or parsley for garnish (optional)

**Instructions:**

1. In a large pot, heat the olive oil over medium heat. Add the chopped onion, diced carrots, and diced celery. Sauté until the vegetables are softened, about 5-7 minutes.
2. Add the minced garlic and grated ginger to the pot, stirring for an additional 1-2 minutes until fragrant.
3. Stir in the ground turmeric, ground cumin, ground coriander, and cayenne pepper, coating the vegetables in the spices.
4. Add the red lentils, vegetable broth, and diced tomatoes (including their juice) to the pot. Bring the mixture to a boil, then reduce the heat to low, cover, and simmer for 20-25 minutes or until the lentils are tender.

5. Stir in the chopped kale and cook for an additional 5 minutes until the kale is wilted.
6. Remove the pot from heat and add the lemon juice. Season the soup with salt and pepper to taste, adjusting as needed.
7. Ladle the anti-inflammatory turmeric soup into bowls and garnish with fresh cilantro or parsley if desired.
8. Serve the soup hot as a nourishing and comforting meal.

## Vegetable Quinoa Soup

**Ingredients:**

- 1 cup quinoa, rinsed and drained
- 1 tablespoon olive oil
- 1 onion, finely chopped
- 2 carrots, peeled and diced
- 2 celery stalks, diced
- 3 cloves garlic, minced
- 1 teaspoon dried thyme
- 1 teaspoon ground cumin
- 1/2 teaspoon paprika
- 6 cups vegetable broth
- 1 can (14 ounces) diced tomatoes

- 1 zucchini, diced
- 1 cup green beans, trimmed and chopped
- 1 cup corn kernels (fresh, frozen, or canned)
- Salt and pepper to taste
- Fresh parsley for garnish (optional)
- Lemon wedges for serving (optional)

**Instructions:**

1. In a large pot, heat the olive oil over medium heat. Add the chopped onion, diced carrots, and diced celery. Sauté until the vegetables are softened, about 5-7 minutes.
2. Add the minced garlic, dried thyme, ground cumin, and paprika to the pot. Stir for an additional 1-2 minutes until the spices are fragrant.
3. Pour in the vegetable broth, diced tomatoes (including their juice), and rinsed quinoa. Bring the mixture to a boil, then reduce the heat to low, cover, and simmer for 15 minutes.
4. Add the diced zucchini, chopped green beans, and corn kernels to the pot. Continue simmering for an additional 10-15 minutes or until the quinoa is cooked and the vegetables are tender.

5. Season the vegetable quinoa soup with salt and pepper to taste. Adjust the seasoning as needed.
6. Ladle the soup into bowls and garnish with fresh parsley if desired.
7. Serve the soup hot, optionally with a squeeze of lemon for added brightness.
8. Enjoy this hearty and nutritious vegetable quinoa soup as a satisfying meal.

## Lentil and Spinach Soup

**Ingredients:**

- 1 cup dried green or brown lentils, rinsed and drained
- 1 tablespoon olive oil
- 1 onion, finely chopped
- 2 carrots, peeled and diced
- 2 celery stalks, diced
- 3 cloves garlic, minced
- 1 teaspoon ground cumin
- 1 teaspoon ground coriander
- 1/2 teaspoon smoked paprika
- 6 cups vegetable broth
- 1 can (14 ounces) diced tomatoes
- 1 cup fresh spinach, chopped

- Juice of 1 lemon
- Salt and pepper to taste
- Fresh parsley for garnish (optional)

**Instructions:**

1. In a large pot, heat the olive oil over medium heat. Add the chopped onion, diced carrots, and diced celery. Sauté until the vegetables are softened, about 5-7 minutes.
2. Add the minced garlic, ground cumin, ground coriander, and smoked paprika to the pot. Stir for an additional 1-2 minutes until the spices are fragrant.
3. Add the rinsed lentils, vegetable broth, and diced tomatoes (including their juice) to the pot. Bring the mixture to a boil, then reduce the heat to low, cover, and simmer for 20-25 minutes or until the lentils are tender.
4. Stir in the chopped fresh spinach and cook for an additional 5 minutes until the spinach is wilted.
5. Remove the pot from heat and add the lemon juice. Season the lentil and spinach soup with salt and pepper to taste, adjusting as needed.
6. Ladle the soup into bowls and garnish with fresh parsley if desired.

7. Serve the soup hot as a wholesome and nourishing meal.

## Chicken and Brown Rice Soup

**Ingredients:**
- 1 tablespoon olive oil
- 1 onion, finely chopped
- 2 carrots, peeled and diced
- 2 celery stalks, diced
- 3 cloves garlic, minced
- 1 teaspoon dried thyme
- 1 teaspoon dried rosemary
- 1 cup brown rice, uncooked
- 6 cups chicken broth
- 1 pound boneless, skinless chicken breasts, diced
- Salt and pepper to taste
- 1 cup frozen peas
- 1 cup corn kernels (fresh, frozen, or canned)
- Juice of 1 lemon
- Fresh parsley for garnish (optional)

**Instructions:**

1. In a large pot, heat the olive oil over medium heat. Add the chopped onion, diced carrots, and diced celery. Sauté until the vegetables are softened, about 5-7 minutes.
2. Add the minced garlic, dried thyme, and dried rosemary to the pot. Stir for an additional 1-2 minutes until the herbs are fragrant.
3. Add the uncooked brown rice to the pot and stir to coat the rice with the vegetables and herbs.
4. Pour in the chicken broth and bring the mixture to a boil. Once boiling, reduce the heat to low, cover, and simmer for 30-40 minutes or until the brown rice is tender.
5. In a separate skillet, cook the diced chicken with a pinch of salt and pepper until fully cooked and no longer pink in the center.
6. Add the cooked chicken, frozen peas, and corn kernels to the pot. Continue simmering for an additional 10 minutes until the vegetables are heated through.
7. Stir in the lemon juice and season the chicken and brown rice soup with salt and pepper to taste. Adjust the seasoning as needed.

8. Ladle the soup into bowls and garnish with fresh parsley if desired.
9. Serve the soup hot as a hearty and satisfying meal.

## Tomato Basil Soup with Chickpeas

**Ingredients:**
- 2 tablespoons olive oil
- 1 onion, chopped
- 2 carrots, peeled and diced
- 2 celery stalks, diced
- 3 cloves garlic, minced
- 2 cans (28 ounces each) whole peeled tomatoes
- 4 cups vegetable broth
- 1 can (15 ounces) chickpeas, drained and rinsed
- 1 teaspoon dried basil
- 1/2 teaspoon dried oregano
- 1/2 teaspoon dried thyme
- Salt and pepper to taste
- 1/2 cup fresh basil, chopped (for garnish)
- Grated Parmesan cheese for serving (optional)

**Instructions:**

1. In a large pot, heat the olive oil over medium heat. Add the chopped onion, diced carrots, and diced celery. Sauté until the vegetables are softened, about 5-7 minutes.
2. Add the minced garlic and cook for an additional 1-2 minutes until fragrant.
3. Pour in the whole peeled tomatoes and vegetable broth. Use a spoon to break up the tomatoes into smaller pieces.
4. Add the drained and rinsed chickpeas to the pot, along with the dried basil, dried oregano, and dried thyme. Stir to combine.
5. Bring the soup to a boil, then reduce the heat to low, cover, and simmer for 20-25 minutes to allow the flavors to meld.
6. Season the tomato basil soup with salt and pepper to taste. Adjust the seasoning as needed.
7. Ladle the soup into bowls and garnish with chopped fresh basil.
8. Optionally, serve the tomato basil soup with a sprinkle of grated Parmesan cheese.
9. Enjoy this comforting and flavorful soup as a light meal or starter.

# Mushroom Barley Soup

**Ingredients:**

- 2 tablespoons olive oil
- 1 onion, finely chopped
- 2 carrots, peeled and diced
- 2 celery stalks, diced
- 3 cloves garlic, minced
- 8 ounces (about 227g) cremini mushrooms, sliced
- 8 ounces (about 227g) button mushrooms, sliced
- 1 cup pearl barley, rinsed and drained
- 8 cups vegetable or mushroom broth
- 1 teaspoon dried thyme
- 1 bay leaf
- Salt and pepper to taste
- Fresh parsley for garnish (optional)

**Instructions:**

1. In a large pot, heat the olive oil over medium heat. Add the chopped onion, diced carrots, and diced celery. Sauté until the vegetables are softened, about 5-7 minutes.

2. Add the minced garlic and sliced mushrooms to the pot. Cook for an additional 5 minutes until the mushrooms release their moisture and start to brown.
3. Stir in the pearl barley and coat it with the vegetables and mushrooms.
4. Pour in the vegetable or mushroom broth and add the dried thyme and bay leaf. Bring the mixture to a boil.
5. Once boiling, reduce the heat to low, cover the pot, and simmer for 45-50 minutes or until the barley is tender.
6. Season the mushroom barley soup with salt and pepper to taste. Remove the bay leaf.
7. Ladle the soup into bowls and garnish with fresh parsley if desired.
8. Serve the soup hot as a hearty and satisfying meal.

## Sweet Potato and Ginger Soup

**Ingredients:**
- 2 tablespoons olive oil
- 1 onion, chopped
- 3 cloves garlic, minced

- 1 tablespoon fresh ginger, grated
- 2 pounds (about 4 medium-sized) sweet potatoes, peeled and diced
- 4 cups vegetable broth
- 1 teaspoon ground cumin
- 1/2 teaspoon ground coriander
- 1/2 teaspoon ground cinnamon
- 1/4 teaspoon cayenne pepper (adjust to taste)
- Salt and pepper to taste
- 1 can (14 ounces) coconut milk
- Juice of 1 lime
- Fresh cilantro for garnish (optional)

**Instructions:**

1. In a large pot, heat the olive oil over medium heat. Add the chopped onion and sauté until softened, about 5 minutes.
2. Add the minced garlic and grated ginger to the pot. Stir for an additional 1-2 minutes until fragrant.
3. Add the diced sweet potatoes to the pot and stir to combine with the onion, garlic, and ginger.
4. Pour in the vegetable broth, ground cumin, ground coriander, ground cinnamon, and cayenne pepper. Bring the mixture to a boil.

5. Once boiling, reduce the heat to low, cover the pot, and simmer for 15-20 minutes or until the sweet potatoes are tender.
6. Use an immersion blender to puree the soup until smooth. Alternatively, transfer the soup to a blender in batches, being cautious with hot liquids.
7. Season the sweet potato and ginger soup with salt and pepper to taste.
8. Stir in the coconut milk and lime juice. Simmer for an additional 5 minutes to allow the flavors to meld.
9. Taste the soup and adjust the seasonings if needed.
10. Ladle the soup into bowls and garnish with fresh cilantro if desired.
11. Serve the sweet potato and ginger soup hot as a comforting and flavorful meal.

## Broccoli and Cheddar Soup

**Ingredients:**
- 2 tablespoons unsalted butter
- 1 onion, chopped
- 2 carrots, peeled and diced

- 2 celery stalks, diced
- 3 cloves garlic, minced
- 1/4 cup all-purpose flour
- 4 cups vegetable or chicken broth
- 4 cups fresh broccoli florets
- 2 cups milk (whole or 2%)
- 2 cups shredded sharp cheddar cheese
- Salt and pepper to taste
- 1/4 teaspoon ground nutmeg
- 1/2 teaspoon dried thyme
- 1/2 cup heavy cream (optional, for added richness)
- Chopped chives or green onions for garnish (optional)

**Instructions:**

1. In a large pot, melt the unsalted butter over medium heat. Add the chopped onion, diced carrots, and diced celery. Sauté until the vegetables are softened, about 5-7 minutes.
2. Add the minced garlic and cook for an additional 1-2 minutes until fragrant.
3. Sprinkle the all-purpose flour over the vegetables and stir to coat, creating a roux. Cook for 2-3 minutes to remove the raw flour taste.

4. Gradually pour in the vegetable or chicken broth, stirring constantly to avoid lumps. Bring the mixture to a simmer.
5. Add the fresh broccoli florets to the pot and continue simmering for 10-15 minutes or until the broccoli is tender.
6. Using an immersion blender, puree the soup until smooth. Alternatively, transfer the soup to a blender in batches, being cautious with hot liquids.
7. Return the pureed soup to the pot and place it over low heat. Stir in the milk, shredded sharp cheddar cheese, salt, pepper, ground nutmeg, and dried thyme. Continue stirring until the cheese is melted and the soup is heated through.
8. If desired, add heavy cream for added richness and stir until well combined.
9. Taste the soup and adjust the seasonings if needed.
10. Ladle the broccoli and cheddar soup into bowls and garnish with chopped chives or green onions if desired.
11. Serve the soup hot as a comforting and cheesy meal.

# Cauliflower and Leek Soup

**Ingredients:**

- 2 tablespoons olive oil
- 2 leeks, white and light green parts only, sliced
- 1 onion, chopped
- 3 cloves garlic, minced
- 1 large head cauliflower, chopped into florets
- 4 cups vegetable broth
- 1 teaspoon ground cumin
- 1/2 teaspoon ground coriander
- 1/2 teaspoon dried thyme
- Salt and pepper to taste
- 4 cups water (or more broth, if preferred)
- 1 cup whole milk or unsweetened almond milk
- Juice of 1 lemon
- Fresh chives for garnish (optional)

**Instructions:**

1. In a large pot, heat the olive oil over medium heat. Add the sliced leeks and chopped onion. Sauté until softened, about 5-7 minutes.
2. Add the minced garlic and cook for an additional 1-2 minutes until fragrant.

3. Add the cauliflower florets to the pot, along with the vegetable broth, ground cumin, ground coriander, dried thyme, salt, and pepper. Pour in enough water to cover the cauliflower.
4. Bring the mixture to a boil, then reduce the heat to low, cover the pot, and simmer for 20-25 minutes or until the cauliflower is tender.
5. Use an immersion blender to puree the soup until smooth. Alternatively, transfer the soup to a blender in batches, being cautious with hot liquids.
6. Return the pureed soup to the pot and place it over low heat. Stir in the whole milk or almond milk and heat through.
7. Add the lemon juice to the soup and stir to combine.
8. Taste the soup and adjust the seasonings if needed.
9. Ladle the cauliflower and leek soup into bowls and garnish with fresh chives if desired.
10. Serve the soup hot as a creamy and flavorful meal.

# Bean and Vegetable Minestrone

**Ingredients:**

- 2 tablespoons olive oil
- 1 onion, finely chopped
- 2 carrots, peeled and diced
- 2 celery stalks, diced
- 3 cloves garlic, minced
- 1 zucchini, diced
- 1 yellow squash, diced
- 1 red bell pepper, diced
- 1 can (15 ounces) cannellini beans, drained and rinsed
- 1 can (15 ounces) kidney beans, drained and rinsed
- 1 can (14 ounces) diced tomatoes
- 1/2 cup small pasta (e.g., ditalini or small shells)
- 8 cups vegetable broth
- 2 teaspoons dried Italian herbs (oregano, basil, thyme)
- Salt and pepper to taste
- 2 cups fresh spinach or kale, chopped
- Grated Parmesan cheese for serving (optional)
- Fresh basil for garnish (optional)

**Instructions:**

1. In a large pot, heat the olive oil over medium heat. Add the chopped onion, diced carrots, and diced celery. Sauté until the vegetables are softened, about 5-7 minutes.
2. Add the minced garlic and cook for an additional 1-2 minutes until fragrant.
3. Stir in the diced zucchini, yellow squash, and red bell pepper. Cook for an additional 5 minutes, allowing the vegetables to soften.
4. Add the drained cannellini beans, kidney beans, diced tomatoes (including their juice), small pasta, and vegetable broth to the pot.
5. Stir in the dried Italian herbs, salt, and pepper. Bring the mixture to a boil, then reduce the heat to low, cover, and simmer for 15-20 minutes or until the pasta is cooked.
6. Add the chopped fresh spinach or kale to the pot and stir until wilted.
7. Taste the minestrone and adjust the seasonings if needed.
8. Ladle the bean and vegetable minestrone into bowls and serve hot.

9. Optionally, garnish with grated Parmesan cheese and fresh basil for added flavor.
10. Enjoy this hearty and nutritious bean and vegetable minestrone as a satisfying meal.

## Spinach and Cannellini Bean Soup

**Ingredients:**

- 2 tablespoons olive oil
- 1 onion, finely chopped
- 2 carrots, peeled and diced
- 2 celery stalks, diced
- 3 cloves garlic, minced
- 2 cans (15 ounces each) cannellini beans, drained and rinsed
- 6 cups vegetable broth
- 1 teaspoon dried thyme
- 1 teaspoon dried rosemary
- Salt and pepper to taste
- 1 bay leaf
- 1 can (14 ounces) diced tomatoes
- 4 cups fresh spinach, chopped
- Juice of 1 lemon
- Grated Parmesan cheese for serving (optional)

**Instructions:**
1. In a large pot, heat the olive oil over medium heat. Add the chopped onion, diced carrots, and diced celery. Sauté until the vegetables are softened, about 5-7 minutes.
2. Add the minced garlic and cook for an additional 1-2 minutes until fragrant.
3. Add the drained cannellini beans, vegetable broth, dried thyme, dried rosemary, salt, pepper, and bay leaf to the pot. Stir to combine.
4. Bring the mixture to a boil, then reduce the heat to low, cover, and simmer for 15-20 minutes.
5. Stir in the diced tomatoes (including their juice) and continue simmering for an additional 10 minutes.
6. Add the chopped fresh spinach to the pot and stir until wilted.
7. Remove the pot from heat and discard the bay leaf.
8. Stir in the lemon juice and taste the soup, adjusting the seasonings if needed.
9. Ladle the spinach and cannellini bean soup into bowls.

10. Optionally, serve with a sprinkle of grated Parmesan cheese for added flavor.
11. Enjoy this delicious and wholesome spinach and cannellini bean soup as a nutritious meal.

## Chicken and Vegetable Ginger Soup

**Ingredients:**
- 1 tablespoon sesame oil
- 1 onion, finely chopped
- 2 carrots, peeled and sliced
- 2 celery stalks, sliced
- 1 red bell pepper, diced
- 3 cloves garlic, minced
- 1 tablespoon fresh ginger, grated
- 1 pound boneless, skinless chicken breasts, thinly sliced
- 8 cups chicken broth
- 1 tablespoon soy sauce
- 1 tablespoon rice vinegar
- 1 tablespoon fish sauce
- 1 teaspoon Sriracha sauce (adjust to taste)
- 1 cup broccoli florets
- 1 cup snow peas, ends trimmed
- 4 ounces rice noodles or vermicelli

- Salt and pepper to taste
- Green onions for garnish
- Fresh cilantro for garnish
- Lime wedges for serving

**Instructions:**

1. In a large pot, heat the sesame oil over medium heat. Add the chopped onion, sliced carrots, sliced celery, and diced red bell pepper. Sauté until the vegetables are softened, about 5-7 minutes.
2. Add the minced garlic and grated fresh ginger to the pot. Stir for an additional 1-2 minutes until fragrant.
3. Add the thinly sliced chicken breasts to the pot and cook until they are no longer pink in the center.
4. Pour in the chicken broth, soy sauce, rice vinegar, fish sauce, and Sriracha sauce. Bring the mixture to a simmer.
5. Add the broccoli florets and snow peas to the pot. Simmer for an additional 5-7 minutes until the vegetables are tender-crisp.

6. Meanwhile, cook the rice noodles or vermicelli according to the package instructions. Drain and set aside.
7. Season the chicken and vegetable ginger soup with salt and pepper to taste. Adjust the seasoning as needed.
8. To serve, place a portion of cooked rice noodles in each bowl and ladle the hot soup over them.
9. Garnish the soup with sliced green onions, fresh cilantro, and lime wedges.
10. Serve the chicken and vegetable ginger soup hot as a flavorful and comforting meal.

## STEWS

### Chicken and Kale Stew

**Ingredients:**
- 1.5 pounds boneless, skinless chicken thighs, cut into bite-sized pieces
- Salt and pepper to taste
- 2 tablespoons olive oil
- 1 onion, finely chopped
- 3 cloves garlic, minced
- 2 carrots, peeled and diced

- 2 celery stalks, diced
- 1 teaspoon dried thyme
- 1 teaspoon dried rosemary
- 1/2 teaspoon smoked paprika
- 1/4 teaspoon red pepper flakes (optional, for heat)
- 4 cups chicken broth
- 1 can (14 ounces) diced tomatoes
- 1 cup quinoa, rinsed and drained
- 1 bunch kale, stems removed and leaves chopped
- Juice of 1 lemon
- Fresh parsley for garnish (optional)

**Instructions:**

1. Season the chicken pieces with salt and pepper.
2. In a large pot, heat olive oil over medium-high heat. Add the seasoned chicken and cook until browned on all sides. Remove the chicken from the pot and set aside.
3. In the same pot, add chopped onion, minced garlic, diced carrots, and diced celery. Sauté until the vegetables are softened, about 5-7 minutes.

4. Stir in dried thyme, dried rosemary, smoked paprika, and red pepper flakes (if using). Cook for an additional 1-2 minutes until the herbs are fragrant.
5. Return the browned chicken to the pot.
6. Pour in chicken broth, diced tomatoes (including their juice), and rinsed quinoa. Bring the mixture to a boil, then reduce the heat to low, cover, and simmer for 15-20 minutes or until the quinoa is cooked.
7. Add the chopped kale to the pot and stir until wilted.
8. Squeeze in the lemon juice and stir to combine.
9. Taste the stew and adjust the seasonings if needed.
10. Ladle the chicken and kale stew into bowls and garnish with fresh parsley if desired.
11. Serve the stew hot as a hearty and nutritious meal.

## Lentil and Sweet Potato Stew

**Ingredients:**
- 2 tablespoons olive oil
- 1 onion, finely chopped

- 3 cloves garlic, minced
- 2 carrots, peeled and diced
- 2 celery stalks, diced
- 2 sweet potatoes, peeled and diced
- 1 cup dry green or brown lentils, rinsed and drained
- 1 teaspoon ground cumin
- 1 teaspoon ground coriander
- 1/2 teaspoon smoked paprika
- 1/4 teaspoon cayenne pepper (adjust to taste)
- 6 cups vegetable broth
- 1 can (14 ounces) diced tomatoes
- 1 bay leaf
- Salt and pepper to taste
- 4 cups fresh spinach or kale, chopped
- Juice of 1 lemon
- Fresh cilantro for garnish (optional)

**Instructions:**

1. In a large pot, heat the olive oil over medium heat. Add the chopped onion, minced garlic, diced carrots, and diced celery. Sauté until the vegetables are softened, about 5-7 minutes.

2. Add the diced sweet potatoes to the pot and cook for an additional 5 minutes, allowing them to slightly brown.
3. Stir in the rinsed lentils, ground cumin, ground coriander, smoked paprika, and cayenne pepper. Coat the vegetables and lentils with the spices.
4. Pour in the vegetable broth, diced tomatoes (including their juice), and add the bay leaf. Bring the mixture to a boil.
5. Once boiling, reduce the heat to low, cover the pot, and simmer for 25-30 minutes or until the lentils and sweet potatoes are tender.
6. Season the stew with salt and pepper to taste. Adjust the seasoning as needed.
7. Stir in the chopped fresh spinach or kale and cook until wilted.
8. Squeeze in the lemon juice and stir to combine.
9. Taste the stew and adjust the seasonings if needed.
10. Ladle the lentil and sweet potato stew into bowls and garnish with fresh cilantro if desired.
11. Serve the stew hot as a flavorful and satisfying meal.

## Turkey and Bean Chili

**Ingredients:**

- 1 tablespoon olive oil
- 1 onion, finely chopped
- 3 cloves garlic, minced
- 1 pound ground turkey
- 2 teaspoons ground cumin
- 2 teaspoons chili powder
- 1 teaspoon smoked paprika
- 1/2 teaspoon dried oregano
- 1/4 teaspoon cayenne pepper (adjust to taste)
- Salt and pepper to taste
- 1 can (15 ounces) black beans, drained and rinsed
- 1 can (15 ounces) kidney beans, drained and rinsed
- 1 can (14 ounces) diced tomatoes
- 1 can (6 ounces) tomato paste
- 2 cups chicken broth
- 1 bell pepper, diced
- 1 cup frozen corn kernels
- Fresh cilantro for garnish (optional)
- Shredded cheddar cheese for topping (optional)
- Sour cream for serving (optional)

**Instructions:**

1. In a large pot, heat the olive oil over medium heat. Add the chopped onion and minced garlic. Sauté until the onion is softened, about 5 minutes.
2. Add the ground turkey to the pot and cook until browned, breaking it apart with a spoon.
3. Stir in the ground cumin, chili powder, smoked paprika, dried oregano, cayenne pepper, salt, and pepper. Cook for an additional 2-3 minutes to toast the spices.
4. Add the drained and rinsed black beans, kidney beans, diced tomatoes (including their juice), tomato paste, and chicken broth to the pot. Stir to combine.
5. Bring the chili to a simmer, then reduce the heat to low, cover, and cook for 20-25 minutes to allow the flavors to meld.
6. Add the diced bell pepper and frozen corn to the pot. Continue simmering for an additional 10-15 minutes until the vegetables are tender.
7. Taste the chili and adjust the seasonings if needed.

8. Ladle the turkey and bean chili into bowls and garnish with fresh cilantro if desired.
9. Optionally, top each serving with shredded cheddar cheese and serve with a dollop of sour cream.
10. Enjoy this hearty and flavorful turkey and bean chili as a satisfying meal.

## Fish and Vegetable Stew

**Ingredients:**

- 1.5 pounds white fish filets (e.g., cod, tilapia), cut into chunks
- Salt and pepper to taste
- 2 tablespoons olive oil
- 1 onion, finely chopped
- 3 cloves garlic, minced
- 2 carrots, peeled and diced
- 2 celery stalks, diced
- 1 bell pepper, diced
- 1 zucchini, diced
- 1 can (14 ounces) diced tomatoes
- 4 cups vegetable broth
- 1 teaspoon dried thyme
- 1 teaspoon dried oregano

- 1/2 teaspoon smoked paprika
- 1 bay leaf
- 1/2 cup dry white wine (optional)
- Juice of 1 lemon
- Fresh parsley for garnish (optional)

**Instructions:**
1. Season the fish chunks with salt and pepper.
2. In a large pot, heat the olive oil over medium heat. Add the chopped onion, minced garlic, diced carrots, diced celery, diced bell pepper, and diced zucchini. Sauté until the vegetables are softened, about 5-7 minutes.
3. Add the fish chunks to the pot and cook until they start to turn opaque.
4. Stir in the diced tomatoes (including their juice), vegetable broth, dried thyme, dried oregano, smoked paprika, and bay leaf. If using, pour in the dry white wine.
5. Bring the stew to a simmer, then reduce the heat to low, cover, and cook for 15-20 minutes to allow the flavors to meld.
6. Squeeze in the lemon juice and stir to combine.
7. Taste the stew and adjust the seasonings if needed.

8. Ladle the fish and vegetable stew into bowls and garnish with fresh parsley if desired.
9. Serve the stew hot as a light and flavorful meal.

## Cabbage and White Bean Stew

**Ingredients:**

- 2 tablespoons olive oil
- 1 onion, finely chopped
- 3 cloves garlic, minced
- 1 small head cabbage, thinly sliced
- 2 carrots, peeled and diced
- 2 celery stalks, diced
- 2 cans (15 ounces each) cannellini beans, drained and rinsed
- 1 can (14 ounces) diced tomatoes
- 4 cups vegetable broth
- 1 teaspoon dried thyme
- 1 teaspoon dried rosemary
- Salt and pepper to taste
- 1 bay leaf
- 1/2 cup dry white wine (optional)
- Juice of 1 lemon
- Fresh parsley for garnish (optional)
- Grated Parmesan cheese for serving (optional)

**Instructions:**

1. In a large pot, heat the olive oil over medium heat. Add the chopped onion and minced garlic. Sauté until the onion is softened, about 5 minutes.
2. Add the thinly sliced cabbage, diced carrots, and diced celery to the pot. Cook for an additional 5-7 minutes until the vegetables start to soften.
3. Stir in the drained cannellini beans, diced tomatoes (including their juice), vegetable broth, dried thyme, dried rosemary, salt, pepper, and bay leaf. If using, pour in the dry white wine.
4. Bring the stew to a simmer, then reduce the heat to low, cover, and cook for 20-25 minutes to allow the flavors to meld.
5. Squeeze in the lemon juice and stir to combine.
6. Taste the stew and adjust the seasonings if needed.
7. Ladle the cabbage and white bean stew into bowls and garnish with fresh parsley if desired.
8. Optionally, serve with a sprinkle of grated Parmesan cheese for added flavor.
9. Enjoy this hearty and nutritious cabbage and white bean stew as a satisfying meal.

## Mushroom and Barley Stew

**Ingredients:**

- 2 tablespoons olive oil
- 1 onion, finely chopped
- 3 cloves garlic, minced
- 8 ounces (about 227g) cremini mushrooms, sliced
- 8 ounces (about 227g) button mushrooms, sliced
- 1 cup pearl barley, rinsed and drained
- 4 cups vegetable or mushroom broth
- 1 teaspoon dried thyme
- 1 teaspoon dried rosemary
- 1 bay leaf
- Salt and pepper to taste
- 2 carrots, peeled and diced
- 2 celery stalks, diced
- 1 can (14 ounces) diced tomatoes
- 1 tablespoon tomato paste
- 1/2 cup dry red wine (optional)
- Fresh parsley for garnish (optional)

**Instructions:**

1. In a large pot, heat the olive oil over medium heat.

2. Add the chopped onion and minced garlic. Sauté until the onion is softened, about 5 minutes.
3. Add the sliced cremini mushrooms and button mushrooms to the pot. Cook for an additional 5-7 minutes until the mushrooms release their moisture and start to brown.
4. Stir in the pearl barley and coat it with the vegetables and mushrooms.
5. Pour in the vegetable or mushroom broth and add the dried thyme, dried rosemary, bay leaf, salt, and pepper. Bring the mixture to a boil.
6. Once boiling, reduce the heat to low, cover the pot, and simmer for 30-40 minutes or until the barley is tender.
7. Add the diced carrots, diced celery, diced tomatoes (including their juice), and tomato paste to the pot. If using, pour in the dry red wine.
8. Continue simmering the stew for an additional 15-20 minutes until the vegetables are tender.
9. Taste the stew and adjust the seasonings if needed.
10. Remove the bay leaf from the pot.

11. Ladle the mushroom and barley stew into bowls and garnish with fresh parsley if desired.
12. Serve the stew hot as a hearty and flavorful meal.

## Chickpea and Spinach Stew

**Ingredients:**

- 2 tablespoons olive oil
- 1 onion, finely chopped
- 3 cloves garlic, minced
- 1 teaspoon ground cumin
- 1 teaspoon ground coriander
- 1/2 teaspoon smoked paprika
- 1/4 teaspoon cayenne pepper (adjust to taste)
- 2 cans (15 ounces each) chickpeas, drained and rinsed
- 4 cups vegetable broth
- 1 can (14 ounces) diced tomatoes
- 1 bay leaf
- Salt and pepper to taste
- 8 cups fresh spinach, chopped
- Juice of 1 lemon
- Fresh cilantro for garnish (optional)
- Greek yogurt for serving (optional)

**Instructions:**

1. In a large pot, heat the olive oil over medium heat. Add the chopped onion and sauté until softened, about 5 minutes.
2. Add the minced garlic, ground cumin, ground coriander, smoked paprika, and cayenne pepper to the pot. Stir for an additional 1-2 minutes until the spices are fragrant.
3. Stir in the drained chickpeas, vegetable broth, diced tomatoes (including their juice), and bay leaf. Bring the mixture to a boil.
4. Once boiling, reduce the heat to low, cover the pot, and simmer for 20-25 minutes to allow the flavors to meld.
5. Season the stew with salt and pepper to taste. Adjust the seasoning as needed.
6. Add the chopped fresh spinach to the pot and stir until wilted.
7. Squeeze in the lemon juice and stir to combine.
8. Taste the stew and adjust the seasonings if needed.
9. Ladle the chickpea and spinach stew into bowls and garnish with fresh cilantro if desired.

10. Optionally, serve each bowl with a dollop of Greek yogurt for added creaminess.
11. Enjoy this nutritious and flavorful chickpea and spinach stew as a satisfying meal.

## Beef and Vegetable Stew with Turmeric

**Ingredients:**

- 1.5 pounds stewing beef, cut into bite-sized pieces
- Salt and pepper to taste
- 2 tablespoons olive oil
- 1 onion, finely chopped
- 3 cloves garlic, minced
- 2 carrots, peeled and diced
- 2 celery stalks, diced
- 2 potatoes, peeled and diced
- 1 teaspoon ground turmeric
- 1 teaspoon ground cumin
- 1 teaspoon paprika
- 1/2 teaspoon ground coriander
- 4 cups beef broth
- 1 can (14 ounces) diced tomatoes
- 1 bay leaf

- 1 cup green beans, chopped
- 1 cup frozen peas
- Fresh parsley for garnish (optional)

**Instructions:**

1. Season the stewing beef with salt and pepper.
2. In a large pot, heat the olive oil over medium-high heat. Add the seasoned beef and brown on all sides. Remove the beef from the pot and set aside.
3. In the same pot, add chopped onion and minced garlic. Sauté until the onion is softened, about 5 minutes.
4. Stir in the diced carrots, diced celery, and diced potatoes. Cook for an additional 5 minutes until the vegetables start to soften.
5. Return the browned beef to the pot.
6. Add ground turmeric, ground cumin, paprika, and ground coriander to the pot. Stir to coat the meat and vegetables with the spices.
7. Pour in the beef broth, diced tomatoes (including their juice), and add the bay leaf. Bring the mixture to a boil.

8. Once boiling, reduce the heat to low, cover the pot, and simmer for 1.5 to 2 hours or until the beef is tender.
9. Add the chopped green beans and frozen peas to the pot. Simmer for an additional 10-15 minutes until the vegetables are tender.
10. Taste the stew and adjust the seasonings if needed.
11. Remove the bay leaf from the pot.
12. Ladle the beef and vegetable stew into bowls and garnish with fresh parsley if desired.
13. Serve the stew hot as a hearty and flavorful meal.

## Cauliflower and Chickpea Curry Stew

**Ingredients:**
- 1 tablespoon coconut oil or olive oil
- 1 onion, finely chopped
- 3 cloves garlic, minced
- 1 tablespoon fresh ginger, grated
- 1 teaspoon ground turmeric
- 1 teaspoon ground cumin
- 1 teaspoon ground coriander
- 1/2 teaspoon cayenne pepper (adjust to taste)

- 1 cauliflower, cut into florets
- 2 cans (15 ounces each) chickpeas, drained and rinsed
- 1 can (14 ounces) diced tomatoes
- 1 can (14 ounces) coconut milk
- 1 cup vegetable broth
- Salt and pepper to taste
- 2 cups spinach or kale, chopped
- Juice of 1 lemon
- Fresh cilantro for garnish (optional)
- Cooked basmati rice for serving

**Instructions:**

1. In a large pot, heat the coconut oil or olive oil over medium heat. Add the chopped onion and sauté until softened, about 5 minutes.
2. Add the minced garlic, grated fresh ginger, ground turmeric, ground cumin, ground coriander, and cayenne pepper to the pot. Stir for an additional 1-2 minutes until the spices are fragrant.
3. Add the cauliflower florets to the pot and coat them with the spice mixture.

4. Stir in the drained chickpeas, diced tomatoes (including their juice), coconut milk, and vegetable broth. Bring the mixture to a boil.
5. Once boiling, reduce the heat to low, cover the pot, and simmer for 15-20 minutes or until the cauliflower is tender.
6. Season the curry stew with salt and pepper to taste. Adjust the seasoning as needed.
7. Add the chopped spinach or kale to the pot and stir until wilted.
8. Squeeze in the lemon juice and stir to combine.
9. Taste the curry stew and adjust the seasonings if needed.
10. Ladle the cauliflower and chickpea curry stew over cooked basmati rice.
11. Garnish with fresh cilantro if desired.
12. Serve the curry stew hot as a flavorful and satisfying meal.

## Tomato and Eggplant Stew

**Ingredients:**
- 2 tablespoons olive oil
- 1 onion, finely chopped
- 3 cloves garlic, minced

- 1 eggplant, diced
- 2 zucchinis, diced
- 1 red bell pepper, diced
- 1 can (14 ounces) diced tomatoes
- 1 can (6 ounces) tomato paste
- 1 teaspoon dried oregano
- 1 teaspoon dried basil
- 1/2 teaspoon dried thyme
- Salt and pepper to taste
- Pinch of red pepper flakes (optional, for heat)
- 1 cup vegetable broth
- Fresh basil for garnish (optional)
- Grated Parmesan cheese for serving (optional)

**Instructions:**

1. In a large pot, heat the olive oil over medium heat. Add the chopped onion and sauté until softened, about 5 minutes.
2. Add the minced garlic to the pot and stir for an additional 1-2 minutes until fragrant.
3. Add the diced eggplant, diced zucchinis, and diced red bell pepper to the pot. Cook for about 7-10 minutes until the vegetables start to soften.
4. Stir in the diced tomatoes (including their juice) and tomato paste. Mix well.

5. Add the dried oregano, dried basil, dried thyme, salt, pepper, and red pepper flakes (if using) to the pot. Stir to combine.
6. Pour in the vegetable broth and bring the mixture to a simmer.
7. Once simmering, reduce the heat to low, cover the pot, and cook for 20-25 minutes or until the vegetables are tender.
8. Taste the stew and adjust the seasonings if needed.
9. Ladle the tomato and eggplant stew into bowls.
10. Optionally, garnish with fresh basil and serve with grated Parmesan cheese for added flavor.
11. Enjoy this flavorful and comforting tomato and eggplant stew as a delicious meal.

## Black Bean and Quinoa Stew

**Ingredients:**

- 1 tablespoon olive oil
- 1 onion, finely chopped
- 3 cloves garlic, minced
- 1 red bell pepper, diced
- 1 green bell pepper, diced

- 1 jalapeño pepper, seeded and minced (optional, for heat)
- 1 cup quinoa, rinsed and drained
- 2 cans (15 ounces each) black beans, drained and rinsed
- 1 can (14 ounces) diced tomatoes
- 1 teaspoon ground cumin
- 1 teaspoon chili powder
- 1/2 teaspoon smoked paprika
- 4 cups vegetable broth
- Salt and pepper to taste
- Juice of 1 lime
- Fresh cilantro for garnish (optional)
- Avocado slices for serving (optional)

**Instructions:**

1. In a large pot, heat the olive oil over medium heat. Add the chopped onion, minced garlic, diced red bell pepper, diced green bell pepper, and minced jalapeño pepper (if using). Sauté until the vegetables are softened, about 5-7 minutes.
2. Add the quinoa to the pot and stir to combine with the vegetables.

3. Stir in the drained black beans, diced tomatoes (including their juice), ground cumin, chili powder, smoked paprika, and vegetable broth. Bring the mixture to a boil.
4. Once boiling, reduce the heat to low, cover the pot, and simmer for 15-20 minutes or until the quinoa is cooked and the stew has thickened.
5. Season the black bean and quinoa stew with salt and pepper to taste. Adjust the seasoning as needed.
6. Squeeze in the lime juice and stir to combine.
7. Taste the stew and adjust the seasonings if needed.
8. Ladle the black bean and quinoa stew into bowls.
9. Optionally, garnish with fresh cilantro and serve with avocado slices for added creaminess.
10. Enjoy this protein-packed and flavorful black bean and quinoa stew as a satisfying meal.

## Chicken and Butternut Squash Stew

**Ingredients:**

- 1.5 pounds boneless, skinless chicken thighs, cut into bite-sized pieces

- Salt and pepper to taste
- 2 tablespoons olive oil
- 1 onion, finely chopped
- 3 cloves garlic, minced
- 1 butternut squash, peeled, seeded, and diced
- 2 carrots, peeled and sliced
- 2 celery stalks, sliced
- 1 teaspoon dried thyme
- 1 teaspoon dried rosemary
- 1/2 teaspoon ground cinnamon
- 4 cups chicken broth
- 1 can (14 ounces) diced tomatoes
- 1 bay leaf
- 1 cup green beans, chopped
- 1 cup frozen peas
- Fresh parsley for garnish (optional)

**Instructions:**

1. Season the chicken pieces with salt and pepper.
2. In a large pot, heat the olive oil over medium-high heat. Add the seasoned chicken and brown on all sides. Remove the chicken from the pot and set aside.

3. In the same pot, add chopped onion and minced garlic. Sauté until the onion is softened, about 5 minutes.
4. Stir in the diced butternut squash, sliced carrots, and sliced celery. Cook for an additional 5 minutes until the vegetables start to soften.
5. Return the browned chicken to the pot.
6. Add dried thyme, dried rosemary, ground cinnamon, chicken broth, diced tomatoes (including their juice), and the bay leaf. Bring the mixture to a boil.
7. Once boiling, reduce the heat to low, cover the pot, and simmer for 30-40 minutes or until the chicken is cooked through and the vegetables are tender.
8. Add the chopped green beans and frozen peas to the pot. Simmer for an additional 10-15 minutes until the vegetables are tender.
9. Taste the stew and adjust the seasonings if needed.
10. Remove the bay leaf from the pot.
11. Ladle the chicken and butternut squash stew into bowls.
12. Optionally, garnish with fresh parsley.

13. Serve the stew hot as a hearty and flavorful meal.

## Vegetarian Gumbo

**Ingredients:**

- 1/2 cup vegetable oil
- 1/2 cup all-purpose flour
- 1 large onion, finely chopped
- 1 green bell pepper, finely chopped
- 2 celery stalks, finely chopped
- 3 cloves garlic, minced
- 1 can (14 ounces) diced tomatoes
- 1 can (14 ounces) tomato sauce
- 1 teaspoon dried thyme
- 1 teaspoon dried oregano
- 1 teaspoon smoked paprika
- 1/2 teaspoon cayenne pepper (adjust to taste)
- Salt and pepper to taste
- 4 cups vegetable broth
- 1 bay leaf
- 1 cup okra, sliced
- 1 can (15 ounces) red kidney beans, drained and rinsed
- 1 cup corn kernels (fresh or frozen)

- 1 cup chopped collard greens or spinach
- 1 tablespoon hot sauce (optional, for extra heat)
- Cooked rice for serving
- Chopped green onions for garnish (optional)

**Instructions:**

1. In a large pot, make a roux by combining vegetable oil and flour over medium heat. Stir constantly until the roux turns a deep brown color. Be careful not to burn it.
2. Add chopped onion, green bell pepper, celery, and minced garlic to the roux. Cook, stirring occasionally, until the vegetables are softened, about 5-7 minutes.
3. Stir in diced tomatoes, tomato sauce, dried thyme, dried oregano, smoked paprika, cayenne pepper, salt, and pepper. Cook for an additional 5 minutes.
4. Pour in vegetable broth and add the bay leaf. Bring the mixture to a boil.
5. Once boiling, reduce the heat to low, cover the pot, and simmer for 20-25 minutes to allow the flavors to meld.

6. Add sliced okra, red kidney beans, corn kernels, and chopped collard greens or spinach to the pot. Continue simmering for an additional 10-15 minutes until the vegetables are tender.
7. If using, add hot sauce for extra heat. Taste the gumbo and adjust the seasonings if needed.
8. Remove the bay leaf from the pot.
9. Ladle the vegetarian gumbo over cooked rice in serving bowls.
10. Optionally, garnish with chopped green onions.
11. Serve the gumbo hot as a flavorful and satisfying meal.

"I am mindful of the positive impact my diet has on my overall health."

"I am on a journey of healing, and my food choices support that journey."

# CHAPTER 10: SMOOTHIES

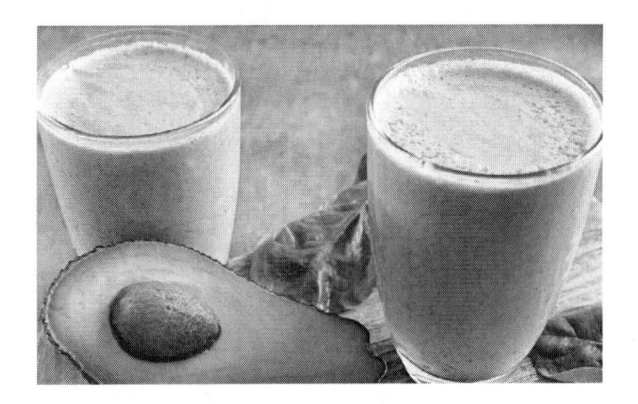

## Tropical Paradise Smoothie

**Ingredients:**

- 1 cup pineapple chunks (fresh or frozen)
- 1/2 cup mango chunks (fresh or frozen)
- 1 banana, peeled and sliced (fresh or frozen)
- 1/2 cup coconut milk
- 1/2 cup orange juice
- 1/2 cup Greek yogurt (optional, for creaminess)
- 1 tablespoon chia seeds (optional, for added nutrition)
- Ice cubes (optional, for a colder smoothie)

**Instructions:**

1. If using fresh fruit, peel and chop the pineapple, mango, and banana.

2. In a blender, combine pineapple chunks, mango chunks, sliced banana, coconut milk, orange juice, Greek yogurt (if using), and chia seeds (if using).
3. Optionally, add ice cubes to the blender for a colder smoothie.
4. Blend the ingredients on high speed until smooth and creamy.
5. Taste the smoothie and adjust the sweetness or thickness by adding more fruit, coconut milk, or orange juice as needed.
6. Once satisfied with the consistency and flavor, pour the tropical paradise smoothie into glasses.
7. Optionally, garnish with additional fruit slices or a sprinkle of chia seeds.
8. Serve the smoothie immediately and enjoy the refreshing taste of the tropical paradise.

## Anti-Inflammatory Turmeric Smoothie

**Ingredients:**

- 1 cup frozen pineapple chunks
- 1 cup frozen mango chunks
- 1 banana, peeled and sliced (fresh or frozen)

- 1 cup coconut water or almond milk
- 1/2 teaspoon ground turmeric
- 1/2 teaspoon ground ginger
- 1 tablespoon chia seeds
- 1 tablespoon flaxseeds
- 1 tablespoon honey or maple syrup (optional, for sweetness)
- Ice cubes (optional, for a colder smoothie)

**Instructions:**

1. If using fresh fruit, peel and chop the banana, and measure out the frozen pineapple and mango chunks.
2. In a blender, combine frozen pineapple chunks, frozen mango chunks, sliced banana, coconut water or almond milk, ground turmeric, ground ginger, chia seeds, flaxseeds, and honey or maple syrup (if using).
3. Optionally, add ice cubes to the blender for a colder smoothie.
4. Blend the ingredients on high speed until smooth and creamy.
5. Taste the smoothie and adjust the sweetness or thickness by adding more honey or maple syrup, coconut water, or almond milk as needed.

6. Once satisfied with the consistency and flavor, pour the anti-inflammatory turmeric smoothie into glasses.
7. Optionally, garnish with a sprinkle of ground turmeric or chia seeds.
8. Serve the smoothie immediately and enjoy the refreshing and anti-inflammatory benefits.

## Protein-Packed Peanut Butter Banana Smoothie

**Ingredients:**
- 1 banana, peeled and sliced (fresh or frozen)
- 1 cup milk (dairy or plant-based)
- 2 tablespoons peanut butter (natural or unsweetened)
- 1/2 cup Greek yogurt
- 1 scoop vanilla protein powder
- 1 tablespoon chia seeds
- 1 tablespoon honey or maple syrup (optional, for sweetness)
- Ice cubes (optional, for a colder smoothie)

**Instructions:**
1. If using a fresh banana, peel and slice it.

2. In a blender, combine banana slices, milk, peanut butter, Greek yogurt, vanilla protein powder, chia seeds, and honey or maple syrup (if using).
3. Optionally, add ice cubes to the blender for a colder smoothie.
4. Blend the ingredients on high speed until smooth and creamy.
5. Taste the smoothie and adjust the sweetness or thickness by adding more honey or maple syrup, milk, or peanut butter as needed.
6. Once satisfied with the consistency and flavor, pour the protein-packed peanut butter banana smoothie into glasses.
7. Optionally, drizzle a bit of peanut butter on top for extra flavor.
8. Serve the smoothie immediately and enjoy the delicious and protein-rich blend.

## Avocado and Spinach Smoothie

**Ingredients:**
- 1 ripe avocado, peeled and pitted
- 2 cups fresh spinach leaves
- 1 banana, peeled and sliced (fresh or frozen)

- 1 cup almond milk or any milk of your choice
- 1/2 cup Greek yogurt
- 1 tablespoon chia seeds
- 1 tablespoon honey or maple syrup (optional, for sweetness)
- Ice cubes (optional, for a colder smoothie)

**Instructions:**

1. In a blender, combine the ripe avocado, fresh spinach leaves, sliced banana, almond milk (or your preferred milk), Greek yogurt, chia seeds, and honey or maple syrup (if using).
2. Optionally, add ice cubes to the blender for a colder smoothie.
3. Blend the ingredients on high speed until smooth and creamy.
4. Taste the smoothie and adjust the sweetness or thickness by adding more honey or maple syrup, milk, or avocado as needed.
5. Once satisfied with the consistency and flavor, pour the avocado and spinach smoothie into glasses.
6. Optionally, garnish with a few spinach leaves or a sprinkle of chia seeds.

7. Serve the smoothie immediately and enjoy the creamy and nutrient-packed goodness.

## Golden Mango Turmeric Smoothie

**Ingredients:**

- 1 cup frozen mango chunks
- 1 banana, peeled and sliced (fresh or frozen)
- 1 cup coconut water or almond milk
- 1/2 teaspoon ground turmeric
- 1/4 teaspoon ground cinnamon
- 1/2 teaspoon fresh ginger, grated
- 1 tablespoon chia seeds
- 1 tablespoon flaxseeds
- 1 tablespoon honey or maple syrup (optional, for sweetness)
- Ice cubes (optional, for a colder smoothie)

**Instructions:**

1. If using fresh banana, peel and slice it. Measure out the frozen mango chunks.
2. In a blender, combine frozen mango chunks, banana slices, coconut water or almond milk, ground turmeric, ground cinnamon, grated fresh ginger, chia seeds, flaxseeds, and honey or maple syrup (if using).

3. Optionally, add ice cubes to the blender for a colder smoothie.
4. Blend the ingredients on high speed until smooth and creamy.
5. Taste the smoothie and adjust the sweetness or thickness by adding more honey or maple syrup, coconut water, or almond milk as needed.
6. Once satisfied with the consistency and flavor, pour the golden mango turmeric smoothie into glasses.
7. Optionally, garnish with a sprinkle of ground turmeric or chia seeds.
8. Serve the smoothie immediately and savor the tropical and anti-inflammatory blend.

## Basil Berry Delight Smoothie

**Ingredients:**

- 1 cup mixed berries (strawberries, blueberries, raspberries)
- 1/2 cup fresh basil leaves, packed
- 1 banana, peeled and sliced (fresh or frozen)
- 1 cup almond milk or any milk of your choice
- 1/2 cup Greek yogurt
- 1 tablespoon chia seeds

- 1 tablespoon honey or maple syrup (optional, for sweetness)
- Ice cubes (optional, for a colder smoothie)

**Instructions:**

1. If using fresh banana, peel and slice it. Measure out the mixed berries.
2. In a blender, combine mixed berries, fresh basil leaves, banana slices, almond milk (or your preferred milk), Greek yogurt, chia seeds, and honey or maple syrup (if using).
3. Optionally, add ice cubes to the blender for a colder smoothie.
4. Blend the ingredients on high speed until smooth and creamy.
5. Taste the smoothie and adjust the sweetness or thickness by adding more honey or maple syrup, milk, or berries as needed.
6. Once satisfied with the consistency and flavor, pour the basil berry delight smoothie into glasses.
7. Optionally, garnish with a fresh basil leaf or a few extra berries.
8. Serve the smoothie immediately and relish the unique combination of basil and berries.

# Pineapple Mint Citrus Smoothie

**Ingredients:**

- 1 cup pineapple chunks (fresh or frozen)
- 1 orange, peeled and segmented
- 1/2 lime, juiced
- 1/4 cup fresh mint leaves, packed
- 1 banana, peeled and sliced (fresh or frozen)
- 1 cup coconut water or water
- 1 tablespoon chia seeds
- 1 tablespoon honey or maple syrup (optional, for sweetness)
- Ice cubes (optional, for a colder smoothie)

**Instructions:**

1. If using a fresh banana, peel and slice it. Prepare the pineapple chunks, orange segments, and fresh mint leaves.
2. In a blender, combine pineapple chunks, orange segments, lime juice, fresh mint leaves, banana slices, coconut water (or water), chia seeds, and honey or maple syrup (if using).
3. Optionally, add ice cubes to the blender for a colder smoothie.
4. Blend the ingredients on high speed until smooth and refreshing.

5. Taste the smoothie and adjust the sweetness or thickness by adding more honey or maple syrup, lime juice, or pineapple as needed.
6. Once satisfied with the consistency and flavor, pour the pineapple mint citrus smoothie into glasses.
7. Optionally, garnish with a sprig of fresh mint or a slice of lime.
8. Serve the smoothie immediately and enjoy the tropical and citrusy goodness.

## Chia Seed and Berry Smoothie

**Ingredients:**

- 1 cup mixed berries (strawberries, blueberries, raspberries)
- 1 banana, peeled and sliced (fresh or frozen)
- 1 cup almond milk or any milk of your choice
- 2 tablespoons chia seeds
- 1 tablespoon honey or maple syrup (optional, for sweetness)
- 1/2 teaspoon vanilla extract
- Ice cubes (optional, for a colder smoothie)

**Instructions:**
1. If using a fresh banana, peel and slice it. Measure out the mixed berries.
2. In a blender, combine mixed berries, banana slices, almond milk (or your preferred milk), chia seeds, honey or maple syrup (if using), and vanilla extract.
3. Optionally, add ice cubes to the blender for a colder smoothie.
4. Blend the ingredients on high speed until smooth and creamy.
5. Taste the smoothie and adjust the sweetness or thickness by adding more honey or maple syrup, milk, or berries as needed.
6. Once satisfied with the consistency and flavor, pour the chia seed and berry smoothie into glasses.
7. Optionally, garnish with a few extra berries or a sprinkle of chia seeds.
8. Serve the smoothie immediately and enjoy the nutrient-packed goodness.

# Creamy Almond Butter Date Smoothie

**Ingredients:**

- 2 tablespoons almond butter
- 4-5 dates, pitted and chopped
- 1 banana, peeled and sliced (fresh or frozen)
- 1 cup almond milk or any milk of your choice
- 1/2 teaspoon vanilla extract
- 1 tablespoon chia seeds
- Ice cubes (optional, for a colder smoothie)

**Instructions:**

1. If using a fresh banana, peel and slice it. Pit and chop the dates.
2. In a blender, combine almond butter, chopped dates, banana slices, almond milk (or your preferred milk), vanilla extract, and chia seeds.
3. Optionally, add ice cubes to the blender for a colder smoothie.
4. Blend the ingredients on high speed until smooth and creamy.
5. Taste the smoothie and adjust the sweetness or thickness by adding more dates, vanilla extract, almond butter, or milk as needed.

6. Once satisfied with the consistency and flavor, pour the creamy almond butter date smoothie into glasses.
7. Optionally, garnish with a drizzle of almond butter or a sprinkle of chopped dates.
8. Serve the smoothie immediately and enjoy the rich and nutty flavor with a hint of natural sweetness.

## Beetroot and Berry Smoothie

**Ingredients:**

- 1 medium-sized beetroot, peeled and chopped
- 1 cup mixed berries (strawberries, blueberries, raspberries)
- 1 banana, peeled and sliced (fresh or frozen)
- 1 cup coconut water or water
- 1 tablespoon chia seeds
- 1 tablespoon honey or maple syrup (optional, for sweetness)
- 1/2 teaspoon ginger, grated (optional, for a zesty kick)
- Ice cubes (optional, for a colder smoothie)

**Instructions:**
1. If using a fresh banana, peel and slice it. Peel and chop the beetroot.
2. In a blender, combine chopped beetroot, mixed berries, banana slices, coconut water (or water), chia seeds, honey or maple syrup (if using), and grated ginger (if using).
3. Optionally, add ice cubes to the blender for a colder smoothie.
4. Blend the ingredients on high speed until smooth and vibrant.
5. Taste the smoothie and adjust the sweetness or thickness by adding more honey or maple syrup, water, or berries as needed.
6. Once satisfied with the consistency and flavor, pour the beetroot and berry smoothie into glasses.
7. Optionally, garnish with a few extra berries or a sprinkle of chia seeds.
8. Serve the smoothie immediately and enjoy the refreshing and nutrient-packed goodness.

# Cucumber Melon Mint Smoothie

**Ingredients:**

- 1 cup cucumber, peeled and diced
- 1 cup melon (cantaloupe or honeydew), diced
- 1 banana, peeled and sliced (fresh or frozen)
- 1/4 cup fresh mint leaves, packed
- 1 cup coconut water or water
- 1 tablespoon chia seeds
- 1 tablespoon honey or maple syrup (optional, for sweetness)
- Juice of 1 lime
- Ice cubes (optional, for a colder smoothie)

**Instructions:**

1. If using a fresh banana, peel and slice it. Peel and dice the cucumber, and prepare the melon by removing the seeds and dicing.
2. In a blender, combine diced cucumber, diced melon, banana slices, fresh mint leaves, coconut water (or water), chia seeds, honey or maple syrup (if using), and the juice of one lime.
3. Optionally, add ice cubes to the blender for a colder smoothie.
4. Blend the ingredients on high speed until smooth and refreshing.

5. Taste the smoothie and adjust the sweetness or thickness by adding more honey or maple syrup, lime juice, or melon as needed.
6. Once satisfied with the consistency and flavor, pour the cucumber melon mint smoothie into glasses.
7. Optionally, garnish with a sprig of fresh mint or a slice of cucumber.
8. Serve the smoothie immediately and enjoy the hydrating and rejuvenating blend.

## Oatmeal Cookie Smoothie

**Ingredients:**

- 1/2 cup old-fashioned rolled oats
- 1 banana, peeled and sliced (fresh or frozen)
- 1/4 cup plain Greek yogurt
- 1 cup almond milk or any milk of your choice
- 1 tablespoon almond butter
- 1 tablespoon honey or maple syrup (optional, for sweetness)
- 1/2 teaspoon ground cinnamon
- 1/4 teaspoon vanilla extract
- Ice cubes (optional, for a colder smoothie)

**Instructions:**

1. In a blender, combine rolled oats, banana slices, Greek yogurt, almond milk (or your preferred milk), almond butter, honey or maple syrup (if using), ground cinnamon, and vanilla extract.
2. Optionally, add ice cubes to the blender for a colder smoothie.
3. Blend the ingredients on high speed until the oats are well incorporated and the smoothie is creamy.
4. Taste the smoothie and adjust the sweetness or thickness by adding more honey or maple syrup, milk, or cinnamon as needed.
5. Once satisfied with the consistency and flavor, pour the oatmeal cookie smoothie into glasses.
6. Optionally, sprinkle a pinch of cinnamon on top for extra flavor.
7. Serve the smoothie immediately and enjoy the wholesome and comforting taste reminiscent of oatmeal cookies.

# CONCLUSION

In conclusion, the "Non-Hodgkin Lymphoma Diet Cookbook: A Complete Guide to Healing" is a comprehensive resource for anyone traversing the difficult journey of Non-Hodgkin Lymphoma. This cookbook goes above and beyond standard recipe collections, providing a holistic approach to nutrition customized exclusively for those receiving treatment and seeking optimal health and recovery.

This cookbook allows readers to make informed food choices that complement their treatment programs by including cancer-fighting dishes and immune-boosting elements. The recipes have been carefully picked to emphasize nutrient-dense, healthy ingredients known for their ability to enhance the body's resilience during cancer treatment.

The emphasis on a well-balanced and nutritious diet emphasizes the necessity of supplying the body with the necessary nutrients for healing and overall well-being.

Individuals with Non-Hodgkin Lymphoma can use this cookbook to find delectable and varied meal alternatives that meet their nutritional needs, ensuring that the culinary component of their journey is a good and healing experience.

In essence, the "Non-Hodgkin Lymphoma Diet Cookbook" is a wonderful companion for those on a healing path, not only giving a multitude of delicious and healthy dishes but also encouraging a sense of empowerment and knowledge. This cookbook exemplifies the transformational power of conscious and purposeful diet in the face of Non-Hodgkin Lymphoma, providing hope and support to individuals and their loved ones throughout the recovery process.

## HAPPY COOKING!

# NON-HODGKIN LYMPHOMA DIET MEAL PLANNER

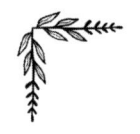

## WEEKLY MEAL PLANNER

| MONDAY | TUESDAY | WEDNESDAY |
|---|---|---|
| | | |

| THURSDAY | FRIDAY |
|---|---|
| | |

**SHOPPING LIST**

| SATURDAY | SUNDAY |
|---|---|
| | |

Notes:

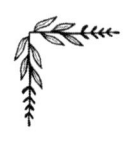

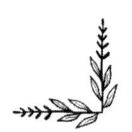

# WEEKLY MEAL PLANNER

| MONDAY | TUESDAY | WEDNESDAY |
|---|---|---|
|  |  |  |

| THURSDAY | FRIDAY |
|---|---|
|  |  |

**SHOPPING LIST**

| SATURDAY | SUNDAY |
|---|---|
|  |  |

Notes:

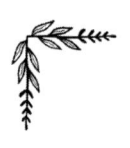

# WEEKLY MEAL PLANNER

| MONDAY | TUESDAY | WEDNESDAY |
|---|---|---|
|  |  |  |

| THURSDAY | FRIDAY | **SHOPPING LIST** |
|---|---|---|
|  |  |  |

| SATURDAY | SUNDAY |
|---|---|
|  |  |

Notes:

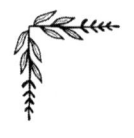

# WEEKLY MEAL PLANNER

| MONDAY | TUESDAY | WEDNESDAY |
|---|---|---|
|  |  |  |

| THURSDAY | FRIDAY | **SHOPPING LIST** |
|---|---|---|
|  |  |  |

| SATURDAY | SUNDAY |
|---|---|
|  |  |

Notes:

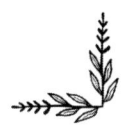

# WEEKLY MEAL PLANNER

| MONDAY | TUESDAY | WEDNESDAY |
|---|---|---|
|  |  |  |

| THURSDAY | FRIDAY |
|---|---|
|  |  |

**SHOPPING LIST**

| SATURDAY | SUNDAY |
|---|---|
|  |  |

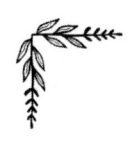

Notes:

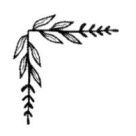

# WEEKLY MEAL PLANNER

| MONDAY | TUESDAY | WEDNESDAY |
|---|---|---|
|  |  |  |

| THURSDAY | FRIDAY |
|---|---|
|  |  |

**SHOPPING LIST**

| SATURDAY | SUNDAY |
|---|---|
|  |  |

Notes:

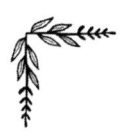

# WEEKLY MEAL PLANNER

| MONDAY | TUESDAY | WEDNESDAY |
|---|---|---|
| | | |

| THURSDAY | FRIDAY |
|---|---|
| | |

**SHOPPING LIST**

| SATURDAY | SUNDAY |
|---|---|
| | |

Notes:

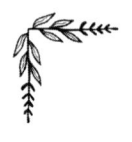

# WEEKLY MEAL PLANNER

| MONDAY | TUESDAY | WEDNESDAY |
|---|---|---|
|  |  |  |

| THURSDAY | FRIDAY |
|---|---|
|  |  |

**SHOPPING LIST**

| SATURDAY | SUNDAY |
|---|---|
|  |  |

Notes:

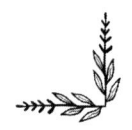

Made in United States
Cleveland, OH
24 March 2025